PRAISE FOR
MOUNTAINS BEYOND MOUNTAINS

"*Mountains Beyond Mountains* is an astonishing book that will leave you questioning your own life and political views. It's the perfect testament to a man who continues to reshape medicine and who has become, undoubtedly, an uncommon savior to a country that desperately needed one. If this book doesn't scream Pulitzer, I don't know what does."

—*USA Today*

"A tale that inspires, discomforts and provokes."

—*The New York Times*

"If I ever go on a retreat again, this is the kind of book I'd like to take for spiritual reading. . . . [Kidder] knows it is impossible to live like Farmer, but the impossibility is the very thing that can somehow give us life."

—*The Washington Post Book World*

"This sensitive, compelling portrait just might, beyond its educational value and absorbing reading, spur at least some readers to help with the kind of action Farmer has dedicated his life to."

—*San Francisco Chronicle*

"Remind[s] us that we're implicated in all the problems [Farmer is] working to solve . . . His complicated humanity only makes him more like the rest of us in our shortcomings—and leaves us asking why we all aren't a little more like him in our virtues."

—*Newsday*

"[An] extraordinary profile . . . a moving testament to Farmer as tireless country doctor and ferocious public health warrior. It'll fill you equally with wonder and hope."

—*People*

"*Mountains Beyond Mountains* will move you, restore your faith in the ability of one person to make a difference in these increasingly maddening, dispiriting times."

—*The San Diego Union-Tribune*

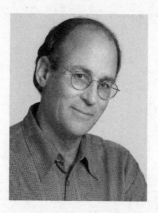

TRACY KIDDER graduated from Harvard, studied at the University of Iowa, and served as an army officer in Vietnam. He has won the Pulitzer Prize, the National Book Award, the Robert F. Kennedy Award, and many other literary prizes. The author of *Home Town, Old Friends, Among Schoolchildren, House,* and *The Soul of a New Machine,* Kidder lives in Massachusetts and Maine.

Mountains

Beyond

Mountains

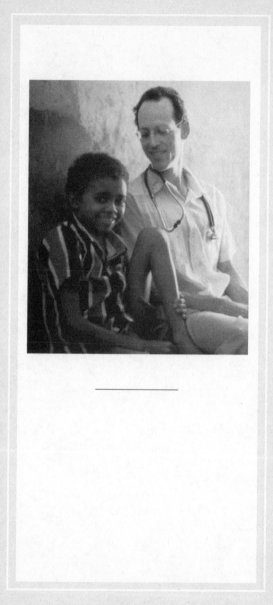

FOR HENRY

AND TIM KIDDER

Dèyè mòn gen mòn.

Beyond mountains there are mountains.

HAITIAN PROVERB

. . . And right action is freedom

From past and future also.

For most of us, this is the aim

Never here to be realised;

Who are only undefeated

Because we have gone on trying . . .

T. S. ELIOT, "THE DRY SALVAGES"

CONTENTS

Part I

—

Doktè Paul

Six years after the fact, Dr. Paul Edward Farmer reminded me, "We met because of a beheading, of all things."

It was two weeks before Christmas 1994, in a market town in the central plateau of Haiti, a patch of paved road called Mirebalais. Near the center of town there was a Haitian army outpost—a concrete wall enclosing a weedy parade field, a jail, and a mustard-colored barracks. I was sitting with an American Special Forces captain, named Jon Carroll, on the building's second-story balcony. Evening was coming on, the town's best hour, when the air changed from hot to balmy and the music from the radios in the rum shops and the horns of the tap-taps passing through town grew loud and bright and the general filth and poverty began to be obscured, the open sewers and the ragged clothing and the looks on the faces of malnourished children and the extended hands of elderly beggars plaintively saying, *"Grangou,"* which means "hungry" in Creole.

I was in Haiti to report on American soldiers. Twenty thousand of them had been sent to reinstate the country's democratically elected government, and to strip away power from the military junta that had deposed it and ruled with great cruelty for three years. Captain Carroll had only eight men, and they were temporarily in charge of keeping the peace among 150,000 Haitians, spread across about one thousand square miles of rural Haiti. A seemingly impossible job, and yet, out here in the central plateau, political violence had all but ended. In the past month, there had been only one murder. Then again, it had been spectacularly grisly. A few weeks back, Captain Carroll's men had fished the headless corpse of the assistant mayor of Mirebalais out of the Artibonite River. He was one of the elected officials being restored to power. Suspicion for his murder had fallen on one of the junta's local functionaries, a rural sheriff named Nerva Juste, a frightening figure to most people in the region. Captain Carroll and his men had brought Juste in for questioning, but they hadn't found any physical evidence or witnesses. So they had released him.

The captain was twenty-nine years old, a devout Baptist from Alabama. I liked him. From what I'd seen, he and his men had been trying earnestly to make improvements in this piece of Haiti, but Washington, which had decreed that this mission would not include "nation-building," had given them virtually no tools for that job. On one occasion, the captain had ordered a U.S. Army medevac flight for a pregnant Haitian woman in distress, and his commanders had reprimanded him for his pains. Up on the balcony of the barracks now, Captain Carroll was fuming about his latest frustration when someone said there was an American out at the gate who wanted to see him.

There were five visitors actually, four of them Haitians. They stood in the gathering shadows in front of the barracks, while their American friend came forward. He told Captain Carroll that his name was Paul Farmer, that he was a doctor, and that he worked in a hospital here, some miles north of Mirebalais.

I remember thinking that Captain Carroll and Dr. Farmer made a mismatched pair, and that Farmer suffered in the comparison. The captain stood about six foot two, tanned and muscular. As usual, a wad of snuff enlarged his lower lip. Now and then he turned his head aside and spat. Farmer was about the same age but much more delicate-looking. He had short black hair and a high waist and long thin arms, and his nose came almost to a point. Next to the soldier, he looked skinny and pale, and for all of that he struck me as bold, indeed downright cocky.

He asked the captain if his team had any medical problems. The captain said they had some sick prisoners whom the local hospital had refused to treat. "I ended up buyin' the medicine myself."

Farmer flashed a smile. "You'll spend less time in Purgatory." Then he asked, "Who cut off the head of the assistant mayor?"

"I don't know for sure," said the captain.

"It's very hard to live in Haiti and not know who cut off someone's head," said Farmer.

A circuitous argument followed. Farmer made it plain he didn't like the American government's plan for fixing Haiti's economy, a plan that would aid business interests but do nothing, in his view, to relieve the suffering of the average Haitian. He clearly believed that the United States had helped to foster the coup—for one thing, by having trained a high official of the junta at the U.S. Army's School of the Americas. Two clear sides existed in Haiti, Farmer said—the forces of repression and the Haitian poor, the vast majority. Farmer was on the side of the poor. But, he told the captain, "it still seems fuzzy which side the American soldiers are on." Locally, part of the fuzziness came from the fact that the captain had released the hated Nerva Juste.

I sensed that Farmer knew Haiti far better than the captain, and that he was trying to impart some important information. The people in this region were losing confidence in the captain, Farmer seemed to be saying, and this was a serious matter, obviously, for a team of nine soldiers trying to govern 150,000 people.

But the warning wasn't entirely plain, and the captain got a little riled up at Farmer's denunciation of the School of the Americas. As for Nerva Juste, he said, "Look, that guy is a bad guy. When I do have him and the evidence, I'll *slam* him." He slapped a fist into his hand. "But I'm not gonna stoop to the level of these guys and make summary arrests."

Farmer replied, in effect, that it made no sense for the captain to apply principles of constitutional law in a country that at the moment had no functioning legal system. Juste was a menace and should be locked up.

So they reached a strange impasse. The captain, who described himself as "a redneck," arguing for due process, and Farmer, who clearly considered himself a champion of human rights, arguing for preventive detention. Eventually, the captain said, "You'd be surprised how many decisions about what I can do here get made in Washington."

And Farmer said, "I understand you're constrained. Sorry if I've been haranguing."

It had grown dark. The two men stood in a square of light from the open barracks door. They shook hands. As the young doctor disappeared into the shadows, I heard him speaking Creole to his Haitian friends.

I stayed with the soldiers for several weeks. I didn't think much about Farmer. In spite of his closing words, I didn't think he understood or cared to sympathize with the captain's problems.

Then by chance I ran into him again, on my way home, on the plane to Miami. He was sitting in first-class. He explained that the flight attendants put him there because he often flew this route and on occasion dealt with medical emergencies on board. The attendants let me sit with him for a while. I had dozens of questions about Haiti, including one about the assistant mayor's murder. The soldiers thought that Voodoo beliefs conferred a special, weird terror on decapitation. "Does cutting off the victim's head have some basis in the history of Voodoo?" I asked.

"It has some basis in the history of brutality," Farmer answered. He frowned, and then he touched my arm, as if to say that we all ask stupid questions sometimes.

I found out more about him. For one thing, he didn't dislike soldiers. "I grew up in a trailer park, and I know which economic class joins the American military." He told me, speaking of Captain Carroll, "You meet these twenty-nine-year-old soldiers, and you realize, Come on, they're not the ones making the bad policies." He confirmed my impression, that he'd visited the captain to warn him. Many of Farmer's patients and Haitian friends had complained about the release of Nerva Juste, saying it proved the Americans hadn't really come to help them. Farmer told me he was driving through Mirebalais and his Haitian friends were teasing him, saying he didn't dare stop and talk to the American soldiers about the murder case, and then the truck got a flat tire right outside the army compound, and he said to his friends, "Aha, you have to listen to messages from angels."

I got Farmer to tell me a little about his life. He was thirty-five. He had graduated from Harvard Medical School and also had a Ph.D. in anthropology from Harvard. He worked in Boston four months of the year, living in a church rectory in a poor neighborhood. The rest of the year he worked without pay in Haiti, mainly doctoring peasants who had lost their land to a hydroelectric dam. He had been expelled from Haiti during the time of the junta but had sneaked back to his hospital. "After the payment," he said, "of an insultingly small bribe."

I looked for him after the plane landed. We talked some more in a coffee shop, and I nearly missed my connecting flight. A few weeks later, I took him to dinner in Boston, hoping he could help make sense of what I was trying to write about Haiti, which he seemed glad to do. He clarified some of the history for me but left me wondering about him. He had described himself as "a poor people's doctor," but he didn't quite fit my preconception of such a person. He clearly liked the fancy restaurant, the heavy cloth napkins, the good bottle of wine. What struck me that evening was how happy he seemed with his life. Obviously, a young man with his advantages could have been doing good works as a doctor while commuting between Boston and a pleasant suburb—not between a room in what I imagined must be a grubby church rectory and the wasteland of central Haiti. The way he talked, it seemed he actually enjoyed living among Haitian peasant farmers. At one point, speaking about medicine, he said, "I don't know why everybody isn't excited by it." He smiled at me, and his face turned bright, not red so much as glowing, a luminescent smile. It affected me quite strongly, like a welcome gladly given, one you didn't have to earn.

But after our dinner I drifted out of touch with him, mainly, I now think, because he also disturbed me. Writing my article about Haiti, I came to share the pessimism of the soldiers I'd stayed with. "I think we should have left Haiti to itself," one of Captain Carroll's men had said to me. "Does it really matter who's in power? They're still gonna have the rich and the poor and no one in between. I don't know what we hope to accomplish. We're still going to have a shitload of Haitians in boats wanting to go to America. But, I guess it's best not even to try and figure it out." The soldiers had come to Haiti and lifted a terror and restored a government, and then they'd left and the country was just about as poor and broken-down as when they had arrived. They had done their best, I thought. They were worldly and tough. They wouldn't cry about things beyond their control.

I felt as though, in Farmer, I'd been offered another way of thinking about a place like Haiti. But his way would be hard to share, because it implied such an extreme definition of a term like "doing one's best."

The world is full of miserable places. One way of living comfortably is not to think about them or, when you do, to send money. Over the next five years, I mailed some small sums to the charity that supported Farmer's hospital in Haiti. He sent back handwritten thank-you notes on each occasion. Once, from a friend of a friend, I heard he was doing something notable in international health, something to do with tuberculosis. I didn't look into the details, though, and I didn't see him again until near the end of 1999. I was the one who made the appointment. He named the place.

CHAPTER 2

Outside the Brigham and Women's Hospital in Boston, you're aware of a relative urban quiet. A Wall Street of medicine surrounds you: the campus of Harvard Medical School and the Countway Medical Library, Children's Hospital, Beth Israel Deaconess, Dana-Farber Cancer Institute, the Brigham. The buildings look imposing packed together, and even awesome when you let yourself imagine what's going on inside. Chest crackings, organ transplants, molecular imagings, genetic probes—gloved hands and machines routinely reaching into bodies and making diagnoses and corrections, so much of human frailty on the one hand and boldness on the other. One feels stilled in the presence of this enterprise. Even the Boston drivers, famously deranged, don't honk much when passing through the neighborhood.

The Brigham occupies one side of Francis Street and envelops, like a city around a Roman ruin, the renovated Victorian lobby of the old Peter Bent Brigham, a relic of the history of Boston medicine. The modern entrance, a towering atrium with marble floors, lies a quarter of a mile away, at the end of a shiny corridor called the Pike—short for turnpike—flanked by banks of elevators, clinical departments to the right and left, inpatient wards on floors above, operating rooms below (forty, not counting the ones in obstetrics), dozens of laboratories in all directions, and mortal dramas everywhere. It's a medical mall, a teaching hospital and a full-service hospital and a tertiary care facility, a hospital to which other hospitals forward their most difficult cases.

Crowds move up and down the Pike, in white uniforms and street clothes, carrying bouquets of flowers, trailing the sound of many mingled conversations.

Four floors down in radiology, Dr. Farmer and his team had staked out a quiet spot, an empty windowless room, and were discussing the last of their cases for the day. Farmer had recently turned forty. Perhaps his hair had receded slightly since I'd last seen him, five years ago. He looked a little thinner, too, and was much more formally attired. He wore wire-framed glasses with little round lenses, and a black suit, and a necktie, cinched up tight. He was still spending most of his time in Haiti, but he was also a big-shot Boston doctor now, a professor of both medicine and medical anthropology at Harvard Medical School, and an attending specialist on the Brigham's senior staff. Looking at him, sitting with two of his students, young doctors in white coats, I imagined a nineteenth-century daguerreotype—the austere, august professor of medicine in a stiff high collar and a waistcoat. That impression didn't last.

He and the young doctors discussed a patient who had recently been treated for a parasite in the brain. The man had become hydrocephalic, and the neurosurgeons had implanted a shunt to drain off the fluid. There was no evidence of further infection, but should the patient be treated for one, just to be safe? "What do you think?" Farmer asked his team, and they batted the question around, and Farmer mostly just listened, though it was clear he was in charge.

After a few minutes, the team agreed: they should treat the patient. Then the phone rang. Farmer picked it up and said, "HIV central. How can we help?"

The caller was a female parasitologist, an old close colleague of Farmer's, offering her view on the hydrocephalic patient. "Worm Lady!" Farmer exclaimed. "How are you, pumpkin? Oh, *I'm* fine. Listen, it's scandalous to say, but we don't agree. We want to treat his ass. ID says treat. Love, ID."

These last two lines were a saying of his. I'd heard him use it earlier in the day, and I'd worked it out for myself. *ID* stood for "Infectious Disease," his specialty. And the command was uttered as if in a letter, and generally meant that he wanted to treat a patient at once, rather than wait for further tests. Clearly, he liked the sound of the words. He seemed to be having a very good time, and from the reactions of his students, small smiles and shakes of the head, which they didn't try to hide from him, I figured that none of his sayings or his jokes or his general ebullience was new for today.

This day—a day in mid-December 1999—had so far been quite ordinary, at least by Brigham standards. Farmer and his team had dealt with six cases, each something of a puzzle, except for the next-to-last case of the day, which seemed rather simple. The resident on the team, a young woman, presented the facts to Farmer, reading from her notes: A thirty-five-year-old man (I'll call him Joe). HIV-positive. Smoked a pack of cigarettes a day. Usually drank half a gallon of vodka. Also used cocaine, both intravenously and by inhalation. Recently overdosed on heroin. Had a chronic cough which five days ago increased, became productive—yellow-green sputum but no blood—and was accompanied by deep chest pain. He had lost twenty-six pounds over the last several months. The radiologists reported a possible right lower lobe infiltrate on his chest X ray—possible tuberculosis, they thought.

The tools for uncovering tuberculosis belong to an older era in medicine, and the diagnosis can be tricky, especially in someone with HIV. Certainly, Joe was a likely target for TB. Of all the infections that can come crowding into a person with HIV disease, TB was the most common worldwide. The disease was rare in Boston, indeed throughout the United States, except in the kinds of places where Joe lived—in homeless shelters and jails and on the streets and under bridges. But in spite of his HIV infection, Joe's immune system was still mostly intact. And he didn't have the classic symptoms of TB, which are fever, chills, and night sweats. "He has terrible teeth," said the resident. She added, "He's a nice guy."

Farmer said, "Let's go see the X ray, shall we?"

They went to another room and put Joe's chest X ray up on a

lighted viewing screen, and Farmer stared, for less than a minute, at the spot where the radiologists thought they saw an infiltrate. Then he said, "That's it? It's rather underwhelming."

They headed upstairs, to visit Joe.

Farmer moved through the Brigham in a long-legged stride, making intermittent headway. He'd pause to receive a hug from a nurse's aide, then to exchange quips in Haitian Creole with a janitor. Then his beeper would go off. Answering the page, he'd greet the hospital operator—whichever of the dozen or so came on line—and quickly ask about her blood pressure, or her husband's heart condition, or her mother's diabetes. Then he'd have to stop at a nurses' station to answer an e-mail about a patient, then to answer a question from a cardiologist. Finally, stethoscope around his neck and singing in creative German, "We are the world. We are das Welt," Farmer led the infectious disease team to the patient's door. Then everything slowed down.

Joe lay on his covers, dressed in blue jeans and a T-shirt, a small man with scarred and wiry arms and prominent collarbones. He had an unkempt beard and unruly hair, and when he smiled nervously at the doctors trooping in, I saw he still had most of his teeth but probably wouldn't for long. Farmer introduced himself and the members of his team. Then he sat down at the head of Joe's bed, on a corner of the mattress, folding himself half around Joe in an agile way that made me think of a grasshopper. He leaned over Joe, gazing down at him, pale blue eyes behind little round lenses. For a moment, I thought Farmer might climb into bed with him. He placed a hand on Joe's shoulder instead and stroked it.

"Your X ray looks good. I think it's probably pneumonia. A little bit of pneumonia. Let me ask you, how's your stomach? Do you have any gastritis these days?"

"I'm eatin' everything in sight of me. Everything in front of me I eat."

Farmer smiled. "You need to gain some weight, my friend. You've lost some weight."

"I didn't eat much when I was outside. I didn't eat much at all. Messin' around, doin' this, doin' that."

"Talk to us a little bit. We're in infectious disease, and we don't think it's tuberculosis. Before I say that, though, any exposure to anybody with TB?"

Joe didn't think so, and Farmer said, "I think we should go ahead and make a recommendation that you not be isolated. We're ID, right? ID says hi. I think you don't need to have a negative airflow room and all that."

"Nah. A fella's in a boat by himself, y'know. People come in with masks on their heads and wash their hands all the time."

"Yeah," said Farmer, adding, "but washing the hands is good, though."

This day was the first on which I'd seen him at work, and it seemed to me just then that his part in the case was closed. Fancy specialist is called in to answer a question. For once, it is vanishingly simple, at least for the specialist. He answers it, makes some small talk with the patient, then departs. But Farmer was still sitting on Joe's bed, and he seemed to like it there.

They talked on and on. Judging from the resident's earlier report, she had asked many of the same questions as Farmer. But Joe was responding with greater candor now. He and Farmer talked about Joe's regular doctor, whom Joe liked, and about the fact that Joe had taken antiretroviral medicines for his HIV, but only erratically, Joe confessed, and Farmer explained that he might well have acquired resistance to some of those drugs and probably shouldn't risk taking others until he found himself in a position to take them faithfully. They talked about drugs and alcohol, Farmer warning him against heroin.

"But really the worst ones are alcohol and cocaine. We were saying downstairs during rounds, we were kinda joking around, saying, Well, we should tell him to smoke more marijuana, because that doesn't hurt as much."

"If I smoke marijuana, I'll create an international incident."

"Not in the hospital, Joe." The two men laughed, looking at each other.

They talked about his HIV. "Your immune system's . . . pretty . . . good, you know. Workin' pretty well. That's why I'm a little worried that you're losing weight, you know. Because you're not losing weight on account of HIV, I bet. You're losing weight because you're not eating. Right?"

"Yeah, that's right."

"Yeah," said Farmer softly. The way he stared at Joe's face just then seemed both intent—as if there were no one else in the world—and also focused elsewhere. I thought in his mind he might be watching Joe from a high window, as Joe went about what are known in social work as the activities of daily living, which in his case would mean scoring some narcotics on a corner, then heading off to his favorite bridge or underpass for camping.

In the midst of all this, another person entered the room, a medical student whom Farmer had invited to join him on rounds. Farmer introduced her. Joe had asked all the other doctors where they'd gone to school. Now he asked the newcomer in his Boston accent, "Are you a Hah-vahd graduate, too?"

"Am *I*?" she said. "Yes."

"Wow," said Joe. He turned back to Farmer. "I got some people from high places lookin' at me, huh?"

"She's a hotshot," Farmer said. And the conversation resumed. "So tell us now, Joe, how can we help? Because we know how the system works here. You come in here, you like us, we like you, you're very nice to us, we're very nice to you, and I think you feel like people here treat you right at home."

"I feel kinda lonesome in this room!" said Joe.

"That's true. And we're going to recommend that you get out of this," said Farmer. "So here's my heavy question for you. Heavy but good."

"What you can do for me."

"Yeah!"

"You ain't gonna believe what I'm gonna say. You ain't ready for this," said Joe.

"I've heard it all, my friend."

"I'd like to have an HIV home where I could go to . . ."

Farmer was gazing down at him again. "Yeah."

"Sleep and eat, watch television, watch games. I'd like somewhere I could go where I can drink a six-pack."

"I understand."

"I'd like to go somewhere where I wouldn't get in trouble, maybe have a couple too many beers, as long as I'm doin' what they tell me, and I'm home on time and I don't mess around, y'know."

"Sure."

"And I don't drive everybody crazy, runnin' out the doors and everything, y'know. Somewhere I could maybe even have a bottle of wine for dinner or something."

"Yeah," said Farmer. "I can see your point." He pursed his lips. "So I'll tell you what. I'll look around, and you're going to be here probably a couple of days, and you know I don't think it's that crazy an idea at all, what you said. Is it better to be out on the street using?"

"Freezing to death," added Joe.

"Freezing to death," said Farmer. "Or inside having a six-pack of beer or some wine with dinner? I know what I would want. The other thing is, if you have a place to stay, you could take medicines, if you want to take medicines."

"Yeah," said Joe, dubiously.

=

A few days later on the message board outside the door of the Brigham's social work department, a cryptic handwritten message appeared. It looked like this:

JOE

OUT	IN
cold	warm
their drugs	our drugs
1/2 gal. vodka	6 pack Bud

Beneath this someone had scrawled: "Why do I know Paul Farmer wrote this?"

Friends of Farmer's had found a homeless shelter for Joe, but of course the social workers had reminded Farmer that shelters forbade drinking, and for good reason, too. He was still pleading Joe's case, just to keep his promise, I supposed, not expecting to win the argument.

Farmer was on service at the Brigham on Christmas. He spent part of the day visiting patients outside the hospital. He brought them all presents, including Joe—who got a six-pack of beer, disguised in wrapping paper.

Joe seemed glad to see him, as well as the present. As Farmer was leaving the shelter, he heard Joe say to another resident, just loudly enough to make Farmer wonder if Joe meant for him to overhear, "That guy's a fuckin' saint."

It wasn't the first time Farmer had heard himself called that. When I asked him his reaction, he said that he felt like the thief in Hawthorne's novel *The Marble Faun,* who steals something from a Catholic church and, before making his escape, dips his hand in holy water. "I don't care how often people say, 'You're a saint.' It's not that I mind it. It's that it's inaccurate."

This was seemly, I thought, resisting beatification. But then he told me, "People call me a saint and I think, I have to work harder. Because a saint would be a great thing to be."

I felt a small inner disturbance. It wasn't that the words seemed immodest. I felt I was in the presence of a different person from the one I'd been chatting with a moment ago, someone whose ambitions I hadn't yet begun to fathom.

=

Farmer finished up his service at the Brigham and went to Haiti on New Year's Day 2000. We had an exchange of e-mails. He had sent me a copy of his latest book, *Infections and Inequalities,* a prodigiously foot-noted discourse with case studies of individual patients to illustrate its main themes—the connections between poverty and disease, the maldistribution of medical technologies in the world, and "the im-modest claims of causality" that scholars and health bureaucrats had offered for those phenomena. At times, it seemed that the author could hardly contain his anger. He described giving antibiotics to an impoverished TB patient, then wrote: "When she received them, she soon began to respond—*almost as if she had a treatable infectious disease.*" The Paul Farmer who had written that book didn't seem much like the Paul Farmer who worked at the Brigham. This one was shouting on every page. I wrote to thank him for the book and added that I planned to read his previous two. "I'm reading your oeuvre," I wrote.

By e-mail he replied: "Ah, but that is not my oeuvre. To see my oeuvre you have to come to Haiti."

CHAPTER 3

Farmer had sent a truck, a sturdy four-wheel-drive pickup, to the Port-au-Prince airport, and I was driven north away from the capital on a two-lane paved road. On the other side of the Plaine du Cul-de-Sac, though, at the foot of a wall of mountains, the road turned into something like a dry riverbed, and the truck began pitching and rolling, scaling its way up the cliff—look down over the edge and you saw a boneyard of truck bodies. No one talked much from then on, not even the friendly, chatty Haitians in the front seat.

On maps of Haiti, the road we traveled, National Highway 3, looks like a major thoroughfare, and indeed it is the *gwo wout la,* the only big road across the central plateau, a narrow dirt track, now strewn with boulders, now eroded down to rough bedrock, now, on stretches that must have been muddy back in the rainy season, baked into ruts that seemed designed to torture wheels, hooves, and feet. It wound through arid mountains and villages of wooden huts. It forded several streams. Trucks of various sizes, top-heavy with passengers, swayed in and out of giant potholes, raising clouds of dust, their engines whining in low gear. A more numerous traffic plodded along on starved-looking donkeys and on foot. Here and there beggars stood on the banks of the road, rubbing concave bellies with one hand while holding out inverted straw hats. Here and there boys with hoes smoothed out little patches of roadway, making shows of their diligence, then lifting their hands in the hope of reward. One noticed absences. An oxcart and no ox, only a man pulling it. Scant trees, especially after Mirebalais. No power poles after the town of Péligre.

The trip, of only about thirty-five miles, lasted three hours and seemed longer by far. It was dark when, at the top of another steep and rocky incline, in the village of Cange, the truck's headlights lit up a tall concrete wall, then a gate in the wall and a sign beside it that read ZANMI LASANTE, Creole for "Partners In Health"—on the sign there was also a picture, of four open hands reaching in from the cardinal points of the compass, all the fingers touching. Then the truck turned in at the gate, and the relief of smooth pavement followed. So I felt Farmer's oeuvre before I saw it.

In daylight, in an all but treeless, baked brown landscape, Zanmi Lasante makes a dramatic appearance, like a fortress on its mountain-side, a large complex of concrete buildings, half covered with tropical greenery. Inside the walls, the world turns leafy. Tall trees stand beside courtyards and walkways and walls, artful constructions of concrete and stone, which mount the forested hillside, past an ambulatory clinic and a women's clinic, a general hospital, a large Anglican church, a school, a kitchen that prepares meals for about two thousand people daily, and, near the top, a brand-new building for the treatment of tuberculosis. The medical complex contains two laboratories. There is running water, and you can hear a big generator churning out electricity. The buildings have tiled floors and clean white walls and ceilings, and paintings by Haitian artists, the soothing kind, full of color, which reimagine the tropical paradise that the journals of Christopher Columbus describe.

The morning after I arrived, I followed Farmer on his rounds through this place, for the first of many times. The general routine was always the same. His day begins around dawn, in the lower court-yard beside the ambulatory clinic. At night I would see in the moon-light the shapes of perhaps a hundred people sleeping there on the ground. In the morning, there are twice as many, people of all ages, the women in dresses and head wraps, the older men in straw hats, and many in shoes that are falling apart, all waiting to see a doctor or nurse.

As Farmer comes in through the gate, dressed in his Haiti clothes—black jeans and a T-shirt—a part of the crowd advances on him. An old man who needs money for food, a woman with a letter she wants him to take to the United States, a young man who has been seen by another doctor here but wants to be examined by Farmer and is calling to him, "I have many things I want to discuss with you, Doktè Paul." Mainly, Farmer searches the crowd for people in urgent need. A nurse has already found one of those, a pretty young woman with her hand wrapped in a towel. The nurse calls to Farmer. He walks over, peels back the towel, and looks in at the hand.

"It's gangrene," he says to me. "Smell it."

He gives the nurse instructions for cleaning the wound. His face looks grim as the nurse leads the woman away. "Her hand was injured fifteen days ago. I wonder if she knows what's coming, you know. As if they didn't have enough problems. Even their minor injuries go unattended."

It usually takes him an hour to make his way through the courtyard. He has almost reached the other side when a small, elderly man approaches, takes off his straw hat, and says in Creole, "I am looking for a man named Doktè Paul."

Farmer smiles. "Do you know Doktè Paul, Father?"

"No," says the old man. "But I was told to seek him out."

One of the staff takes the man by the arm. "Let's see if we can find Doktè Paul." As she leads him away toward another doctor, Farmer finally escapes, a lanky figure striding up the shaded concrete path toward the kitchen and the little room above it where every morning, before patients, he sends and receives e-mail via a satellite phone.

=

I may as well say that from the moment I saw Zanmi Lasante, out there in the little village of Cange, in what seemed to me like the end of the earth, in what was in fact one of the poorest parts of the poorest country in the Western Hemisphere, I felt I'd encountered a miracle. In Haiti, I knew, per capita incomes came to a little more than one American dollar a day, less than that in the central plateau. The country had lost most of its forests and a great deal of its soil. It had the worst health statistics in the Western world. And here, in one of the most impoverished, diseased, eroded, and famished regions of Haiti, there was this lovely walled citadel, Zanmi Lasante. I wouldn't have thought it much less improbable if I'd been told it had been brought by spaceship.

My first week in Cange I met a peasant farmer who had brought a sick child to the hospital—by donkey, on a trek of twelve miles along Highway 3. I asked him if he'd felt relieved when he got to Cange and the medical complex. I needn't have bothered. He looked surprised at the question and simply said, "Wi!" There were a handful of other clinics and hospitals in the region, but none were well-equipped and some were downright unsanitary, and everywhere patients had to pay for medicines, and even the gloves that would be used to examine them, and very few people in the central plateau could pay much of anything. At Zanmi Lasante, too, patients were supposed to pay user fees, the equivalent of about eighty American cents for a visit. Haitian colleagues of Farmer's had insisted on this. Farmer was the medical director, but he hadn't argued. Instead—this was often his way, I would learn—he had simply subverted the policy. Every patient had to pay the eighty cents, except for women and children, the destitute, and anyone who was seriously ill. Everyone had to pay, that is, except for almost everyone. And no one—Farmer's rule—could be turned away.

Perhaps a million peasant farmers relied on Zanmi Lasante. At the moment, about a hundred thousand lived in its catchment area, the area served by its community health workers, seventy in all. Some patients came great distances, as distance is measured in a country of ruined roads and villages served only by footpaths—from Port-au-Prince and Haiti's southern peninsula, and from towns along the border with the Dominican Republic, speaking Spanish. Most came from the central plateau, on the battered, overloaded passenger trucks that navigated Highway 3. Many came on foot and by donkey. Now and then out on the road, a bed moved slowly toward the front gate, a bearer at each corner, a patient on the mattress.

Sometimes Zanmi Lasante's pharmacy muddled a prescription or ran out of a drug. Now and then the lab technicians lost a specimen. Seven doctors worked at the complex, not all of them fully competent—the staff was entirely Haitian, and Haitian medical training is mediocre at best. But Zanmi Lasante had built schools and houses and communal sanitation and water systems throughout its catchment area. It had vaccinated all the children, and had greatly reduced both local malnutrition and infant mortality. It had launched programs for women's literacy and for the prevention of AIDS, and in its catchment area had reduced the rate of HIV transmission from mothers to babies to 4 percent—about half the current rate in the United States. A few years back, when Haiti had suffered an outbreak of typhoid resistant to the drugs usually used to treat it, Zanmi Lasante had imported an effective but expensive antibiotic, cleaned up the local water supplies, and stopped the outbreak throughout the central plateau. In Haiti, tuberculosis still killed more adults than any other disease, but no one in Zanmi Lasante's catchment area had died from it since 1988.

The money for Zanmi Lasante was funneled through a small public charity that Farmer had founded—Partners In Health, with headquarters in Boston. The bills were small by American standards. Farmer and his staff of community health workers treated most tuberculosis patients in their huts and spent between $150 and $200 to cure an uncomplicated case. The same cure in the United States, where most TB patients were hospitalized, usually cost between $15,000 and $20,000.

My local hospital in Massachusetts was treating about 175,000 patients a year and had an annual operating budget of $60 million. In 1999 Zanmi Lasante had treated roughly the same number of people, at the medical complex and out in the communities, and had spent about $1.5 million, half of that in the form of donated drugs. Some of the cash came from grants but most of it from private donations, the largest from a Boston developer named Tom White, who had given millions over the years. Farmer contributed, too, though he didn't know exactly how much.

I became aware of the logistical facts of Farmer's life only gradually, so they didn't seem completely unusual until I totaled them up. In 1993 the MacArthur Foundation had given him one of its so-called genius grants—in his case some $220,000. He'd donated the entire sum to Partners In Health, to create a research branch for the organization—the Institute for Health and Social Justice, he called it. He made about $125,000 a year from Harvard and the Brigham, but he never saw his paychecks or the honoraria or royalties, both fairly small sums, that he received for his lectures and writings. The bookkeeper at PIH headquarters cashed the checks, paid his bills—and his mother's mortgage—and put whatever was left in the treasury. One day in 1999, Farmer tried to use his credit card and was told he'd reached his limit, so he called the bookkeeper. She told him, "Honey, you are the hardest-workin' broke man I know."

Back when he was a bachelor, he'd stayed in the basement of Partners In Health headquarters during his sojourns in Boston. Four years ago he'd married a Haitian woman, Didi Bertrand. He saw no reason to change their Boston living quarters, but when their daughter was born, in 1998, his wife insisted it was time to move. Now they had an apartment in Eliot House at Harvard, which they used when in Boston. But they weren't often there. These days, Didi and their two-year-old spent the academic year in Paris, where Didi was finishing her own studies in anthropology. Several friends had told Farmer he should spend more time with them. "But I don't have any patients in Paris," he'd say. It was obvious that he missed his family. When I was with him in Haiti, he called them at least once a day, from the room with the satellite phone. In theory, he spent four months in Boston and the rest of the year in Cange. In fact, those periods were all chopped up, by trips to places where he did have patients. Years ago he'd gotten a letter from American Airlines welcoming him to their million-mile club. He'd traveled at least two million miles since.

He had a small house in Cange, the closest thing in his life to a home, perched on a cliff across the road from the medical complex. It was a modified *ti kay,* a replica of the better sort of peasant house, with a metal roof and concrete floors and exceptional in that it had a bathroom, though without hot water. Many times when I looked inside his house, his bed appeared unused. He told me he slept about four hours a night but a few days later confessed, "I can't sleep. There's always somebody not getting treatment. I can't stand that."

Little sleep, no investment portfolio, no family around, no hot water. On an evening a few days after arriving in Cange, I wondered aloud what compensation he got for these various hardships. He told me, "If you're making sacrifices, unless you're automatically following some rule, it stands to reason that you're trying to lessen some psychic discomfort. So, for example, if I took steps to be a doctor for those who don't have medical care, it could be regarded as a sacrifice, but it could also be regarded as a way to deal with ambivalence." He went on, and his voice changed a little. He didn't bristle, but his tone had an edge: "I feel ambivalent about selling my services in a world where some can't buy them. You *can* feel ambivalent about that, because you *should* feel ambivalent. *Comma.*"

This was for me one of the first of many encounters with Farmer's use of the word *comma,* placed at the end of a sentence. It stood for the word that would follow the comma, which was *asshole.* I understood he wasn't calling me one—he would never do that; he was almost invariably courteous. *Comma* was always directed at third parties, at those who felt comfortable with the current distribution of money and medicine in the world. And the implication, of course, was that you weren't one of those. Were you?

=====

In the mornings, I followed Farmer from the courtyard, to e-mail, and then to his office—on the ground floor of the newest building, the Thomas J. White Tuberculosis Center. Diplomas hung on the wall, together with a photograph of Haiti's first elected president, Jean-Bertrand Aristide—Farmer's friend of many years—posing with a boy whom Farmer had cured of TB. There was an examining table, an X-ray viewer, a desk, and a new office chair that the staff had bought him for Christmas. It still had some tinsel on it.

Farmer sits down at his desk. "Now the objective is?" He looks at me. I shrug. He says, "To stay put. Because people are lurking outside. Lurkaceous behavior."

A crowd of perhaps thirty—on occasion, I counted forty—waits in the hall, some sitting on benches, some milling around. A nurse in white uniform enters, saying to Farmer, indignantly, "I always say patients must sit down, and they don't listen to me."

Farmer smiles at her, making the Haitian hand slap, the back of one hand into the palm of the other. "It's a cross we must carry," he says. The nurse stalks out. He looks over at me. "You can't sympathize with the staff too much, or you risk not sympathizing with the patients."

They are indeed the poor and the maimed and the halt and the blind. An elderly man in treatment for pulmonary TB who makes me think of Ray Charles. (He's blind but wears glasses. He had said he wanted glasses, so Farmer had found him a pair.) A younger man whom Farmer refers to as Lazarus, who arrived some months ago on a bed frame carried by relatives, wasted by AIDS and TB to about 90 pounds, now weighing in at about 150, cured of TB and his AIDS arrested thanks to medications. A healthy-looking young woman whose father, only a month ago, was saving up for her coffin.

And, on the other hand, a lovely-looking young woman being treated for drug-resistant TB, now in the midst of a sickle-cell crisis and moaning in pain. "Okay, *doudou*. Okay, *cherie*," Farmer coos. He orders morphine.

A man with gastritis in late middle age. In Haiti, Farmer told me, that could mean thirty years old, since 25 percent of Haitians die before they reach forty. "It's because there's a near famine here," says Farmer, examining him. "The man is muscular. Perhaps in his declining years he can't scrap for food as well, or maybe there's someone he's trying to feed." He orders nutritional supplements.

A sixteen-year-old boy too weak to walk, who weighs only sixty pounds. Farmer diagnoses an ulcer. "His body's gotten used to starvation. We're gonna buff him up." Farmer hefts a can of the dietary supplement Ensure. "This is good stuff. We'll give him three cans a day. So we'll give him a couple hundred dollars of Ensure, and I'll take great pleasure in violating the principle of cost-efficacy."

A very small, elderly-looking woman, her body bent at the waist, at a right angle. Long before Farmer met her, tuberculosis of the spine had devoured pieces of her backbone—a case of Pott's disease, easily cured but it had gone untreated and was "burnt out." There's nothing to be done for it now. She's come for money and food and company. Farmer stands when she enters, greeting her as *mami mwen,* "my mother." He bends down, practically kneeling, and she kisses him on one cheek, then the other, and says, "A son always cares for his mother." Farmer gets her a chair, and she holds on to it, still standing, resting her chin on the seat, and watches as he ministers to the next several patients.

As at the Brigham, he seems bound to get as close to them as possible. He has them sit in a chair right next to his, so that, I figure, he can get his thin, white, long-fingered hands on them. He calls the older women "Mother," the older men "Father." Many bring him presents. Milk in a green bottle with a corncob stopper. *"Oh, cheri! Mesi anpil, anpil!"*—"Thank you, thank you!" Farmer says. He smiles and, staring at the bottle on his desk, says in English, "Unpasteurized cow's milk in a dirty bottle. I can't wait to drink it." He turns to me. "It's so awful you might as well be cheerful."

I look up. A very pregnant woman is forcing her way past the nurse and in through his office door. She's infected with HIV and is here to receive isoniazid prophylaxsis, having also been exposed to TB. She also needs money for food; her husband has died. She lifts her voice high and cries cheerily, "You guys are all my husbands!" A young man enters next. "Doktè Paul? I came here and was sick. Now I'm much better. So I would like a picture taken."

On the wall beside his desk, Farmer has taped up three sheets of yellow legal paper, on every line a task to be completed, and beside each of those a hand-drawn box, in Creole a *bwat.* I've noticed that if he completes a chore that he forgot to put on the list, he writes down the chore, makes a *bwat* beside it, then puts a check in the box. This seems to give him an inordinate pleasure, and I must admit that I feel some myself, completely unjustified, when he says, "We're getting a lot done."

The list on the wall contains about sixty imperatives—to assemble the slides for upcoming speeches, to get Lazarus a Bible and a pair of nail clippers, to give another patient the wristwatch he bought for him in the Miami airport, to obtain sputum samples from some of the patients with drug-resistant TB and take them to Boston for testing. The list seems to speak of what, in Boston, might be called an interesting practice. Certainly it is varied. One item reads, "Sorcery consult."

In one of his books, Farmer had written that there was a distinction, in the Haitian countryside, between belief in sorcery and "the theories and practices called voodoo." That is, not every peasant practiced the indigenous religion called Voodoo, but virtually everyone, including Catholics and Protestants and Voodooists, believed in the reality of *maji,* of sorcery. For many people around Cange, magic spells sent by enemies were the deep cause of many illnesses. And many people around Cange believed that Farmer, like all good Voodoo priests, knew how to contend with *maji.*

One local peasant told me, speaking of Farmer, "God gives everyone a gift and his gift is healing." Once at a public ceremony, a former patient of his stood up and declared, "I believe he is a god." It was also said around Cange, usually in whispers, "Doktè Paul works with both hands"—that is, both with science and with the magic necessary to remove ensorcellments. Most of the encomiums seemed to embarrass and amuse Farmer. But this last, he's explained, has a painful side. "Haitians believe in sorcery because their culture has evolved in the absence of effective medicine. So of course they believe in sorcery, in sicknesses that someone has sent to them. Why else would someone fall into a coma? And when someone is very sick and people are used to seeing them die with the same symptoms and you give them meds and they rapidly recover, people think. And then they start talking." In his experience, most Haitians eagerly embrace effective medicine. He has dozens of Voodoo priests among his patients, some of them serving as virtual community health workers, bringing him ill parishioners.

Sorcery is, at bottom, the Haitians' way of explaining suffering, but the allegations themselves can cause suffering. Now an elderly woman enters Farmer's office. She's the subject of the sorcery consult. The other day in the courtyard Farmer saw her son moping around and asked him what was wrong. "My mother hates me," he said. In fact, the mother believes her son "sent" the sickness that killed another son. As she sits down beside Farmer and he begins telling her not that sorcery doesn't exist but that he knows sorcery wasn't involved in this instance, she lifts her chin and averts her face. Gradually, she softens. But it will probably take months to reconcile her fully with her surviving son. When she leaves, Farmer says he feels "eighty-six percent amused." And, I suppose this means, 14 percent sad.

The woman had insisted that her son had "sold" his brother, using the Creole word once applied to slaves. (Haitian beliefs in sorcery were perhaps in part inspired by the slave masters' own fears, born of guilt. "A great many beliefs and practices in Haitian magic originate from Normandy, Berry, Picardy or ancient Limousin," writes the anthropologist Alfred Métraux.) Moreover, accusations like the woman's always seem to spring from the jealousies that great scarcity inspires. The accused son lives in a better *ti kay* than his mother. In effect, she was saying this son didn't care about his mother, so he must have been the one who sent sorcery to kill his brother. These kinds of allegations, accusations that arise out of economic inequalities, are common, Farmer says. They can tear families and friends apart. "When I realized that, I thought, Oh, man! It's not enough that the Haitians get destroyed by everything else, but they also have an exquisite openness to being injured by words."

After a few days in Cange with Farmer, I came to expect such interpretive discourses. Farmer called them "narrating Haiti." I don't want to exaggerate this tendency of his. He was capable of maintaining companionable silences, indeed, often seemed to prefer them to talk, and he made light conversation at least as often as he proselytized. Besides, I was trying to get the hang of his cosmology, so I egged him on, sometimes even badgered him into narrating Haiti. When he got going, though, everything around us became the occasion for drawing a moral about the suffering of the Haitian poor, which often also served as a lesson about the suffering of the world's poor. Sometimes he'd pause to ask for a reaction: "You feelin' me?"

And for me the problem often was that I couldn't muster a sufficient response internally. I'd feel sorry that so many Haitian children still died of measles—though not in Zanmi Lasante's catchment area—but I'd also feel that I could never be sorry enough to satisfy him. I'd end up annoyed at Farmer for a time, in the way one gets annoyed at others when one has done them a disservice.

=

Days and nights ran together. Farmer liked to tell his Harvard students that to be a good clinician you must never let a patient know that you have problems too, or that you're in a hurry. "And the rewards are so great for just those simple things!" Of course, this meant that some patients waited most of a day to see him and that he rarely left his office before dark.

Through the louvered windows high on the wall behind his desk, I see stars shivering in the warm night. A sad-faced young man takes his seat beside Farmer and stares down at his own feet, shod in ragged running shoes, splitting at the heels. His name is Ti Ofa. He has AIDS. When he's on duty at the Brigham, Farmer runs the hospital's AIDS service, and he's handled Ti Ofa's case as he would have in Boston, treating various opportunistic infections with antibacterials, until the infections become chronic. Zanmi Lasante doesn't have the wherewithal to measure viral loads and CD4 counts, but from long experience Farmer knows the virus is about to begin its endgame with Ti Ofa, its overwhelming stage. Ti Ofa says, "I feel ashamed."

"Anybody can catch this. I told you that already," Farmer says. He opens a drawer in his desk and takes out a large plastic bottle. It contains indinavir, one of the new protease inhibitors used for treating AIDS.

No one else, not at this time, is treating impoverished Haitians with the new antiretroviral drugs. Indeed, almost no one in any poor country is treating poor people who have the disease. Even some of Farmer's friends in the Haitian medical establishment have told him he's crazy to take on AIDS this way in Cange, and certainly many experts in international health would agree. Leaving aside all other objections, the new AIDS drugs could cost Zanmi Lasante about five thousand dollars a year per patient. Nonetheless, Farmer had started some patients on triple therapy. A few months ago, he gave a speech to a group in Massachusetts called Cambridge Cares About AIDS. "Cambridge cares about AIDS," he told them. "But not nearly enough." He wondered if he'd gone too far, but afterward, at his suggestion, health workers in the audience and people who themselves had AIDS collected a bunch of unused drugs, and he ended up with enough to treat a few more of his patients here in Cange. He intends to increase those numbers, he says. He and his colleagues back in Massachusetts are working on grant proposals to obtain a larger, more reliable supply. They'll find the money, he's told me. "*Of course* we'll find the money."

He holds up the precious bottle for Ti Ofa to see. He shakes it, and the pills rattle around inside. He tells Ti Ofa that he'll start treating him with this drug and two others now. They won't eradicate HIV from his body, Farmer explains, but they will take away his symptoms and, if he's lucky, let him live for many years as if he'd never caught the virus. He only has to promise that he'll never miss a dose.

Ti Ofa says he won't, but he's still looking at his shoes. Farmer leans closer to him. "I don't want you to be discouraged."

Ti Ofa looks up. "Just talking to you makes me feel better. Now I know I'll sleep tonight." He wants to talk, and I suppose he knows he's welcome to do so. "My situation is so bad. I keep hurting my head because I live in such a crowded house. We only have one bed, and I let my children sleep on it, so I have to sleep under the bed, and I forget, and I hit my head when I sit up. I don't forget what you did for me, Doktè Paul. When I was sick and no one would touch me, you used to sit on my bed with your hand on my head. They had to tie up the dogs in the village, you walked around so late to see sick people." Ti Ofa declares, "I would like to give you a chicken or a pig."

Ordinarily Farmer's skin is pale, with a suggestion of freckles underneath. Now it reddens instantly, from the base of his neck to his forehead. "You've already given me a lot. Stop it!"

Ti Ofa smiles. "I am going to sleep well tonight."

"Okay, *neg pa*"—"my man"—says Farmer.

Then it's time for rounds, first by flashlight down the paths to the hospital, and through the dimly lit main ward, where the beds are filled by adults, and then, with trepidation, to the Children's Pavilion upstairs, where there always seems to be a baby with the sticklike limbs, the bloated belly, the reddish hair of kwashiorkor, a form of starvation. Just a week or so ago, on his first morning back in Cange, Farmer had lost a baby to meningitis, in its ghastly *purpura fulminans* presentation, the small vessels bleeding into the baby's skin, making a rash of purple spots. And, only days later, another baby, from beyond Zanmi Lasante's catchment area, died of tetanus.

Farmer lingers beside the crib of a little girl with wasted arms and a torso bloated by pleural effusion—caused by extrapulmonary TB. She lies on her side. He reaches in and strokes her shoulder, saying softly, almost singing, in English, "Michela wants to give up, but we're not going to let her, are we? No, we're not going to let her."

Then he walks back up the hill, to the TB hospital, saving this visit for last, he says, because just now everyone up there is getting better. Most of the patients have gathered in one room and are sitting on the beds watching a soccer game on a wavy, snowy TV screen. "Look at you bourgeois people watching TV!" Farmer says.

The patients laugh. One of the young men looks up at him. "No, Doktè Paul, not bourgeois. If we were bourgeois, we would have an antenna."

"It cheers me up," Farmer says on the way out. "It's not all bad. We're failing on seventy-one levels, but not on one or two." Then it's back down the hill and out the gate and across Highway 3 to his house.

Night in the mostly unelectrified central plateau is vast. Roosters are crowing—they crow here at all hours—and a warm wind rustles the leaves of the trees that surround Farmer's little patio, lit by battery power. It feels like the cabin of a small boat at sea, a cozy enclosure, where Farmer now sets to work on speeches and grant proposals, assisted by a young member of Partners In Health, a PIH-er in Farmer's vernacular, sent from Boston for this purpose.

He holds a huge stack of medical studies on his lap. After a time, he puts them aside. "I'm not into this, guys." He takes me on a survey of his grounds. It's clear that a proper guest has to accompany him. "This is called hortitorture," he says. He recites the names of the trees, vines, shrubs, flowers that he's planted here over the years. I count about forty different species. Finally, in the dim light from the patio, he studies a new fern that has just come up. "It's just vibrant and happy and healthy. The way a patient should be."

The word, *patient,* is like a bell. He goes back to work on the pile of clinical studies. Minutes later Ti Jean, Zanmi Lasante's chief handyman, appears out of the dark, summoning him back across Highway 3.

———

In a bed by the door of the hospital lies a moaning thirteen-year-old girl, just arrived by donkey ambulance. Two young Haitian doctors— one is just an intern—stand beside her bed, eyes half-lowered, lips pursed, as Farmer makes the Haitian hand slap, saying, *"Doktè-m yo, doktè-m yo, sa k'ap pase-n?"*—"Doctors, doctors, what's going on with you?" His voice sounds plaintive, not angry, as he lectures: You do not administer an antibiotic to a person with meningitis until you have done a spinal tap and know the variety of meningitis and thus which drug will work.

Then he does the job himself, the young doctors looking on, holding the girl down.

"I'm very good at spinal taps," he's told me. He seems to be, and besides, he's left-handed, and to my eyes left-handers at work have always looked adroit. The veins stand out on Farmer's thin neck as he eases the needle in. Wild cries erupt from the child: *"Li fe-m mal, mwen grangou!"* Farmer looks up, and for a moment he's narrating Haiti again. "She's crying, 'It hurts, I'm hungry.' Can you believe it? Only in Haiti would a child cry out that she's hungry during a spinal tap."

CHAPTER 4

S oon after I arrived to visit him in Cange, Farmer said he'd be my
Virgil here. I think that, when it came to Haiti, he viewed almost
everyone as a potential subject for education, or reeducation. No
other country in the world had been subjected to as much "idiotic
commentary," he said, and it would have been hard to argue the point,
given the fact that, for instance, the name of Haiti's indigenous religion had long since become the synonym for crazy ideas and sheer
luridness.

Farmer liked to tell a story about his own education in Haiti, a
story about the relation between medicine and beliefs in sorcery. Back
in 1988, a woman from Zanmi Lasante's catchment area had died of
tuberculosis while he was in Boston recovering from a badly broken
leg. When he returned to Cange, several of the staff told him the
woman wouldn't have died if he'd been on hand. They meant this as
a compliment. He converted it to self-reproach. He wanted a medical
system that functioned in his absence. He gave everyone in the
woman's family jobs at Zanmi Lasante and called a series of staff
meetings to figure out what was wrong with their system for treating TB.

The staff had a lively debate. Zanmi Lasante's community health
workers, who lived among the peasant farmers, who had been until
recently mostly peasant farmers themselves, spoke about the economic impediments to treatment, pointing out that the poorest patients tended to fare worst, certainly in part because of malnutrition.

One health worker recited a Haitian saying: "Giving people medicine for TB and not giving them food is like washing your hands and drying them in the dirt." But most of the Haitian professionals on the staff—the doctors, the nurses, the technicians—offered explanations that laid the blame in the minds of the patients, the kinds of explanations one often reads in scholarly journals. Once they felt better but long before they were cured, patients stopped taking their pills, the professionals said, and patients did this in part because they didn't believe TB came from microbes but believed it was sent to them by enemies, via sorcery.

Farmer felt intellectually torn. The health workers' theory amounted to a description of the kind of socioeconomic arrangement that he called "structural violence." But he was also an anthropologist in training, schooled in the importance of the kinds of cultural beliefs that the professionals cited. So he designed a study. He was still a student at Harvard. The study was like a class he created and then attended as a pupil.

He selected two groups of TB patients. During the study, each group got free treatment, the same they would have received at the Brigham. But one group got other services as well, including regular visits from community health workers and small monthly cash stipends for food and child care and transportation to Cange. Farmer hiked to the many villages of the patients, visiting all of them in their huts. This took weeks. "A hundred chatty Haitians," he would say. "Don't try this at home." He asked all of them, among other questions, if they believed TB came from sorcery, and all but a very few in both groups said that they did. And yet, when the results came in, the cure rates for the two groups were dramatically different. Of the patients who had received only free medicine, a mere 48 percent were cured. By contrast, everyone in the group that received the cash stipends and other services made a full recovery. Whether a patient believed that TB came from germs or sorcery didn't seem to have made any difference at all.

Farmer felt puzzled. "I expected to buy into the idea that what's in people's minds affects their behavior and the outcomes," he told me.

And he was at a loss for explanations, until he began reinterviewing the patients and called on one of his favorites, a sweet, rather elderly woman. When he had first interviewed her, about a year before, she'd taken mild offense at his questions about sorcery. She'd been one of the few to deny she believed in it. "Polo, *cheri*," she had said, "I'm not stupid. I know tuberculosis comes from people coughing germs." She'd taken all her medicines. She'd been cured.

But now, a year later, when he asked her again about sorcery, she said that of course she believed in it. "I know who sent me my sickness, and I'm going to get her back," she told him.

"But if you believe that," he cried, "why did you take your medicines?"

She looked at him. He remembered a small sympathetic smile. The smile, he thought, of an elder explaining something to a child— in fact, he was only twenty-nine. *"Cheri,"* she said, *"eske-w pa ka konprann bagay ki pa senp?"* The Creole phrase *pa senp* means "not simple," and implies that a thing is freighted with complexity, usually of a magical sort. So, in free translation, she said to Farmer, "Honey, are you incapable of complexity?"

And then of course it dawned on him that he knew plenty of Americans—he was one himself—who held apparently contradictory beliefs, such as faith in both medicine and prayer. He felt, he said, as though he hung in the air before his patient, "suspended by her sympathy and bemusement."

The study was for him a command—to worry more about his patients' material circumstances than about their beliefs. From then on, all TB patients in the catchment area received the full package of services. Each continued to get what is called directly observed therapy, a community health worker on hand to be sure the patient took the medicines on schedule, and each got the monthly cash stipend—the equivalent of about five American dollars—to pay for extra food, child care, and transportation to a monthly doctor's appointment at Zanmi Lasante. The program had worked well, indeed, couldn't have worked better. They hadn't lost a single patient in twelve years, and Farmer wasn't about to change any of the rules.

Just recently, a TB patient from a village called Morne Michel hadn't shown up for his monthly doctor's appointment. So—this was one of the rules—someone had to go and find him. The annals of international health contain many stories of adequately financed projects that failed because "noncompliant" patients didn't take all their medicines. Farmer said, "The only noncompliant people are physicians. If the patient doesn't get better, it's your own fault. Fix it." A favorite Doktè Paul story in the village of Kay Epin was of the time, many years back, when Farmer had chased a man into a field of cane, calling to him plaintively to come out and let him treat him. He still went after patients occasionally. To inspire the staff, he said, and to give him a break from his office. So he was going to Morne Michel himself, and was taking me with him.

"Beyond mountains there are mountains." The proverb appeared to describe the location of Morne Michel, the most distant of all the settlements in Zanmi Lasante's catchment area. At breakfast on the appointed day, Farmer told the women in the kitchen his intentions. "Ooooo!" they cried. One said, "Morne Michel? Polo, do you want to kill your *blan*?"

She meant me, of course. She wasn't being rude. The women in the kitchen called even Farmer a *blan*—usually they called him *ti blan mwen,* meaning "my little white guy." But a *blan* isn't necessarily white-skinned; one might say, every *blan* becomes white by virtue of being a *blan.* The African American medical student Farmer had brought here some months back, for instance. Some people at Zanmi Lasante had wondered if he was Farmer's brother, and later some had mistaken another visiting black American student of Farmer's for the first one, and when Farmer teased them about this, one of the staff had said— Farmer swore this was true—"All you *blan* look alike."

Farmer drove the first leg in the pickup truck, south down National Highway 3, past two-roomed huts with metal roofs and little granaries on stilts—built, he explained, to keep food safe from animals, but rats still ate about a third of harvests—and stunted-looking pigs and goats and scrawny yellow dogs. Smiling for a moment, he said that Haitian peasants had a lot of sayings: that they're the only farmers with land so steep they break their legs in their cornfields, that their dogs are so skinny they have to lean against trees in order to bark. Soon a reservoir came into view, a mountain lake far below the road. The scene looked beautiful, blue waters set among steep, arid mountainsides. And, if you saw with peasant eyes, Farmer said, the scene looked violent and ugly, a lake that had buried the good farmland and ravaged the highlands.

He parked beside the ruin of a small cement factory. Plants were growing helter-skelter high up on the rusted structure. A hundred yards away stood a concrete buttress dam. These days, when he wasn't in Haiti, he gave a lot of speeches, sometimes several in one day, and in every one I heard, he talked about the dam. It appeared in all the books he had published by 2000 and in the books that he had helped to write and edit, and also in many of his journal articles—forty-two of those by then. As a scholar and writer, Farmer had taken his greatest pains to assert the interconnectedness of the rich and poor parts of the world, and the dam was his favorite case study.

It stops up Haiti's largest river, the Artibonite. It's called the Péligre Dam and the impounded waters behind it, the Lac de Péligre. The U.S. Army Corps of Engineers had planned it. Brown & Root of Texas, among others, built the structure in the mid-1950s during the reign of one of Haiti's American-supported dictators, with money from the U.S. Export-Import Bank. It was advertised as "a development project," and no doubt some of the people behind its creation believed it a gift to Haiti. But no one seems to have given much thought to the peasant farmers who lived in the valley upstream.

The project was intended to improve irrigation and to generate power. It wasn't as though the peasants of the central plateau didn't need and want modern technology, Farmer said. But, as they themselves often remarked, they didn't even get electricity or water for their land. Most didn't get money either. In fact, the dam was meant to benefit agribusinesses downstream, mostly American-owned back then, and also to supply electricity to Port-au-Prince, especially to the homes of the numerically tiny, wealthy Haitian elite and to foreign-owned assembly plants. Since the flooding of the valley, many peasant girls and boys from Cange, children of what Farmer called "the water refugees," had left home looking for work in the capital, where they cooked and cleaned and stitched Mickey Mouse dolls and baseballs, more than a few of them nowadays returning home with AIDS.

When Farmer first saw this piece of Haiti and began to ferret out its history, old-timers talked longingly to him about the days before the water rose, when families lived on farms beside the river and everyone had enough to eat and something left over to sell. Some remembered being warned that their land was going to be submerged. But the river had always flowed by, and they'd examined the dam in progress, and they couldn't believe that a mere wall of concrete could hold back their river. One of the old people of Cange remembered seeing the water rising and suddenly realizing that his house and goats would be underwater in a matter of hours. "So I picked up a child and a goat and started up the hillside." Families had hurried away, carrying whatever they could save of their former lives, turning back now and then to watch the water drown their gardens and rise up the trunks of their mango trees. For most, there was nothing to do but settle in the steep surrounding hills, where farming meant erosion and widespread mal-nutrition, tending nearer every year toward famine. And for years there were wailings and curses and loud arguments among old neigh-bors, fighting over titles to the land that was left.

Things got worse. Even after the dam, most peasants still had their black, low-slung Creole pigs, which they kept like bank accounts, to pay for things such as school tuition. But in the early 1980s, they lost those as well. Alarmed about an outbreak of African swine fever in the Dominican Republic, afraid that it might threaten the American pork industry, the United States led an effort to destroy all the Creole pigs in Haiti. The plan was to replace them with pigs purchased from Iowa farmers. But these were much more delicate, much more expensive to house and feed, and they didn't thrive. Many peasants ended up with no pigs at all. When school started the year after the slaughter, enrollments had declined dramatically, throughout the country and around Cange.

We walked across the top of the dam. The railings were rusted, the concrete flaking. To our right the roiled waters of the Artibonite rushed away, and to our left a few small canoelike vessels plied blue, placid waters. It looked almost like a tropical resort. Farmer walked briskly along. A small juvenile escort followed him for a time. Local people heading the other way smiled when they saw him and said, *"Bonjou, Doc mwen"*—"Good morning, my Doc." There were clouds then sun then clouds again, and a gentle breeze. I felt vigorous and cheered by borrowed popularity.

On the other side of the dam, a footpath—loose dirt and stones—went straight up. Farmer had a slipped disk from eighteen years of traveling Highway 3. His left leg had been surgically repaired after he'd been hit by a car back in 1988, and it turned out at a slight angle—like a kickstand, one of his brothers said. He had congenital high blood pressure and mild asthma, which developed after he'd recovered from a possible case of tuberculosis. But when I got to the top of that first hill, sweating and panting, he was sitting on a rock, writing a letter to an old friend, a contributor to Partners In Health whose spouse had recently died. It was the first of many hills.

We passed smiling children climbing steep rocky paths that I had to clamber up on all fours. They were carrying water, in pails and plastic jugs that once held things like paint, oil, and antifreeze. The full containers must have weighed half as much as the children did, and the children had no shoes. We passed beside many patches of millet, the national staple, which seemed to be growing out of rocks, not soil, and small stands of banana trees and, now and then, other tropical species, Farmer pausing to apply the Latin and familiar names—papaw, soursop, mango—a gloomy litany because there were so many fewer of each variety than there should have been.

On a fair number of the trees that remained in those hills, and also on rocks, I saw political graffiti, usually scrawled in red paint: "Titid" and the number "2001." These were, respectively, the nickname of former President Aristide and the year in which, judging from all the posters and graffiti I had seen around Cange, he would be reelected. Politics, I supposed, was one means by which Haitian peasants avoided hopelessness. Many aid experts from prosperous places gladly expressed hopelessness on the Haitians' behalf, Farmer would say. By this point on our hike, I too was guilty. The houses we passed in the mountains were much worse than most of the ones around Cange. They had dirt floors and roofs made of banana fronds, which, Farmer pointed out, leaked during the rainy season, turning the floors to mud. We passed a group of women who were washing clothes in the rivulet of a gully. "It's Saturday," said Farmer. "Washing day. I guess the Maytag repairman didn't come." Haitians, he said, are a fastidious people. "I know. I've been in all their nooks and crannies. But they blow their noses into dresses because they don't have tissues, wipe their asses with leaves, and have to apologize to their children for not having enough to eat."

"Misery," I said. But this would not suffice. He was on a roll.

"And don't think they don't know it," he said. "There's a WL line— the 'They're poor but they're happy' line. They do have nice smiles and good senses of humor, but that's entirely different."

Like many of his remarks, this one gave me pause.

Just when you thought you had the hang of his worldview, he'd surprise you. He had problems with groups that on the surface would have seemed like allies, that often were allies in fact, with for example what he called "WL's"—white liberals, some of whose most influential spokespeople were black and prosperous. "I love WL's, love 'em to death. They're on our side," he had told me some days ago, defining the term. "But WL's think all the world's problems can be fixed without any cost to themselves. We don't believe that. There's a lot to be said for sacrifice, remorse, even pity. It's what separates us from roaches."

We walked on. I noticed, as I had around Cange, that many people we passed wore clothes from America, brand-name running shoes that had seen much better days and baseball caps and T-shirts bearing the logos of professional sports teams and country clubs. "Kennedys" was the generic name for stuff like that. Back in the 1960s, Farmer had explained, President Kennedy sponsored a program that sent machine oil, among other things, to Haiti. The Haitians tried to use the oil for other purposes, such as cooking, and concluded that the gift was of inferior quality. Ever since, the president's name had been synonymous here with secondhand and shoddy goods. Now and then one saw another kind of import, meant strictly for adornment. There was a young worker at Zanmi Lasante who wore a new-looking, Haitian-style straw hat on which he or his wife had sewn a homemade piece of cloth that read NIKE.

We went on, deeper and deeper into the mountains, Farmer leading the way. We chatted front to back. I was drenched in sweat. I couldn't see even signs of perspiration on his neck—his pencil neck as friends of his called it. Many people waved to him—the lifted hand motionless, the fingers fluctuant, like the legs of insects on their backs. "Do you see how Haitians wave? Don't you love it? You dig?" he said to me, waving back with his fingers. The trail wound across barren, steeply folded mountainsides. I had thought that I was fairly fit, but at the top of every hill, Farmer would be waiting for me, smiling and making excuses for me when I apologized—I was fourteen years older; I wasn't used to the climate.

The one-way trip to Morne Michel usually took him two hours. About three hours after we'd set out, we arrived at the hut of the noncompliant patient, another shack made of rough-sawn palm wood with a roof of banana fronds and a cooking fire of the kind Haitians call "three rocks."

Farmer asked the patient, a young man, if he disliked his TB medicines.

"Are you kidding?" he replied. "I wouldn't be here without them."

It turned out that he'd been given confusing instructions the last time he was in Cange, and he hadn't received the standard cash stipend. He hadn't missed any doses of his TB drugs, however. Good news for Farmer. Mission accomplished. He'd made sure that the patient's cure wasn't being interrupted.

We started back. I slipped and slid down the paths behind Farmer.

"Some people would argue this wasn't worth a five-hour walk," he said over his shoulder. "But you can never invest too much in making sure this stuff works."

"Sure," I said. "But some people would ask, 'How can you expect others to replicate what you're doing here?' What would be your answer to that?"

He turned back and, smiling sweetly, said, "Fuck you."

Then, in a stentorian voice, he corrected himself: "No. I would say, 'The objective is to inculcate in the doctors and nurses the spirit to dedicate themselves to the patients, and especially to having an outcome-oriented view of TB.' " He was grinning, his face alight. He looked very young just then. "In other words, 'Fuck you.' "

We started on again, Farmer saying over his shoulder, "And if it takes five-hour treks or giving patients milk or nail clippers or raisins, radios, watches, then do it. We can spend sixty-eight thousand dollars per TB patient in New York City, but if you start giving watches or radios to patients here, suddenly the international health community jumps on you for creating *nonsustainable* projects. If a patient says, I really need a Bible or nail clippers, well, for God's sake!"

I was scrambling down yet another steep incline when from a copse below I heard a commotion—yelling, then a little lull, then yells again. In a few minutes a cockfighting pit came into view, a corral entirely surrounded, several people deep, by men in straw hats and ragged pants and shirts, shod in torn sneakers, flip-flops, old brown dress shoes without laces. On the periphery, there were a pair of competing food sellers and a couple of men who had set up games of Zo— it involved a board and a thing that looked like a Victorian teapot, for shaking dice. There were also women at the edges of the crowd. A place was made for Farmer at the railing. He watched for a moment. The cocks were circling each other. Then one made a charge, wings flapping, and Farmer turned away.

He moved to the edge of the trees, where suddenly a couple of chairs materialized, metal chairs with torn Naugahyde seats, one red, one blue. This always happened in the countryside when I was with

Farmer, the appearance of chairs, one for Doktè Paul, one for his *blan*. We sat. In a moment, we were surrounded. By women, a dozen or more—elderly-looking women, lovely young women in sundresses with one torn shoulder strap. A middle-aged woman, with a beautiful face but several front teeth missing, leaned against a tree and spoke softly to Farmer. The others stood by other trees or sat in the dirt close by, some speaking to him, too, from time to time. One woman was telling him that they needed an additional community health worker up here, but mostly they were just passing the time. Is there a more widespread notion than the one that rural people are laconic, and is there a rural place anywhere in the world whose people really are?

I was worn out, my clothes completely drenched. My thoughts were wandering. I thought of the chairs we sat on—discarded, I imagined, during the refurbishing of an office in Minneapolis or Miami— and about their long journey here. I imagined I knew why the women were doing this, ignoring the national sport on a Saturday to gather around Farmer and chat with such mild desultoriness, voices low and musical and unhurried. Some years ago he had added to his growing medical program a health project just for women and, lacking a gynecologist on the staff, had made his own quick study of the specialty and for a time practiced it here. He'd probably given a number of these women the first pelvic exams they'd ever received, and had talked to them about birth control, offering it if they wanted. The shouts and cries from the cockpit seemed to be reaching a crescendo, but they sounded far away. I felt as if I could fall asleep, and as if I already had, enfolded in femininity.

The rest of the way back was mostly a descent, but there were still some slopes to climb. I straggled up out of another ravine and as usual found Farmer waiting for me. He stood at the edge of a cliff, gazing out. I walked over to him. The view from where he stood was immense. Scrims of rain and clouds and swaths of sunlight swept across the yellow mountains in front of us and the yellow mountains beyond those mountains and over the Lac de Péligre. The scene, I realized, would have looked picturesque to me before today. So maybe I'd learned something. Not enough to suit Farmer, I suspected. Education wasn't what he wanted to perform on the world, me included. He was after transformation.

I offered him a slightly moist candy, a Life Saver from my pocket. He took it, said, "Pineapple! Which, as you know, is my favorite," and then went back to gazing.

He was staring out at the impounded waters of the Artibonite. They stretched off to the east and west and out of sight among the mountains. From here the amount of land the dam had drowned seemed vast. Still gazing, Farmer said, "To understand Russia, to understand Cuba, the Dominican Republic, Boston, identity politics, Sri Lanka, and Life Savers, you have to be on top of this hill."

The list was clearly jocular. So was his tone of voice. But I had the feeling he had said something important. I thought I got it, generally. This view of drowned farmland, the result of a dam that had made his patients some of the poorest of the poor, was a lens on the world. His lens. Look through it and you'd begin to see all the world's impoverished in their billions and the many linked causes of their misery. In any case, he seemed to think I knew exactly what he meant, and I realized, with some irritation, that I didn't dare say anything just then, for fear of disappointing him.

Part II

—

The Tin Roofs
of Cange

It was impossible to spend any time with Farmer and not wonder how he happened to choose this life. I did some looking in the usual place.

His parents came from western Massachusetts. He was born in the aging mill town of North Adams in 1959, the second of six children, three boys, three girls. His mother, Ginny, was a farmer's daughter. She quit college early to marry. You could see her in him quite clearly. She was fairly tall, and slender. Her nose was his exactly, and her tendency to blush.

Farmer's father—Paul, Sr.—was a big man, about six two, weighing in at between 230 and 250 pounds. He was a fine and ferociously competitive athlete, known as Elbows to people who played basketball with him. In later years his younger daughters would rechristen him the Warden, on account of his strictness—no makeup, no boyfriends, no staying out late. He was a restless sort of man. He had a steady job as a salesman in Massachusetts, but then a friend of his told him there was real money to be made in sales down south in Alabama: "Alabama is a sleeping giant." In 1966 the Warden moved his growing family south to Birmingham.

In retrospect, the years in Alabama were happy ones for Ginny. They were a little short on furniture but lived in a real house, and they bought an automatic washing machine, the first one she'd ever had. The Warden also arranged for economical family vacations by buying, at public auction, a large bus. The bus, oddly enough, had once been used as a mobile TB clinic, and to accommodate an X-ray machine, a turretlike extrusion had been added to its roof. The bus's brand name was Blue Bird. The Blue Bird Inn, the Farmers called it. Meanwhile, Paul, Jr.—P.J. or Pel to his family—was flourishing. His sisters remember him as a scrawny boy, intense in anger and affection. "And," they'd say, "he had this huge brain." The elementary school authorities placed him in a gifted and talented class. In fourth grade he started a herpetology club. He invited all his classmates to the house for the first meeting, and asked Ginny to make Rice Krispies Treats. None of his classmates came, and he was very quiet for a time, a sure sign to his older sister that he was upset. But the family, in effect, became the club, attendance required by the Warden's decree. They'd meet in the living room. P.J. would dress up in a bathrobe and point with a stick at charcoal drawings he'd made of reptiles and amphibians—even his siblings had to admit the pictures were beautiful. He'd discourse on the animals' diets, reproduction, life spans, their interesting and unusual characteristics. He'd always announce each species by its Latin name. A sister remembered thinking, "We should just beat him up and go back out and play." But after a while she and the others would get interested and start asking questions.

Both his grandmothers were devout Roman Catholics, and his family went to church and he went through the rites of first communion and confirmation, even serving as an altar boy for a time, but he didn't feel engaged. "It was perfunctory," he'd remember, "although I liked the Mass itself and still do. But it was nowhere near as exciting as the stuff I was reading." The parents of some fellow students in the gifted and talented class owned a bookstore, and when he was about eleven they gave him a copy of J.R.R. Tolkien's trilogy, *The Lord of the Rings*. He read it all in the space of a couple of days, and immediately read it again. Then he brought the book to the public library and told the woman at the desk, "I want other books like this." She gave him a handful of fantasy novels. He brought them back. "No, this isn't it." That went on for a time, until finally one day the librarian—no doubt with some misgivings; the boy was only eleven years old—handed him a copy of *War and Peace*. "This is it!" he told the librarian about a week later. "This is just like *Lord of the Rings!*" Years afterward he'd say, "I mean, what could be more religious than *Lord of the Rings* or *War and Peace?*"

═

Sales work in Alabama disappointed the Warden. He turned to teaching. But the atmosphere in Birmingham in the latter 1960s made him and Ginny worry for their children's safety. The Warden found a job in a public school in Florida, and so one day in 1971 the family stowed their belongings inside the Blue Bird Inn, all that it would hold. The Warden and Ginny and the children wrestled the washing machine out to the bus, but it wouldn't fit through the side doors. One of Farmer's most vivid memories was of the moment when they pulled away from their rented house in Birmingham. He watched his pretty young mother gaze sadly out the back windows of their bus at the washing machine, white among the bits of coal that littered the backyard. It would be her last washing machine for many years. They headed for Brooksville, a small town north of Tampa near the Gulf Coast.

Farmer's older sister remembered riding in the Blue Bird Inn down the town's fancy street, all overhung with Spanish moss and flanked by houses with antebellum-looking porticoes, and the Warden at the bus's wheel saying, "We'll get a house like one of these." For the time being, though, they drove out to the Brentwood Lake Campground, a trailer park beside a piney woods. The Warden must have been preoccupied. He drove toward the campground office and either forgot about the turret on the roof or didn't see the power wires overhead. In any case, the turret snagged the wires and tore them down.

After the mess was sorted out, the Warden found a concrete block for a front step, and they settled in. Ginny took a cashier's job at a Winn-Dixie supermarket and learned to work the register while smiling at customers and stomping on the pedal that moved the conveyor belt. She was a Winn-Dixie cashier who read *Cry, the Beloved Country* to her children at night and, years later, went to Smith College and got her bachelor's degree. What none of the family remembered from those days in Florida was hearing her complain. "My mother is like the Virgin Mary without the virgin part," one of Farmer's sisters would say. "Loving, kind, nonjudgmental. She was the calm one always." Ginny would remark years later that she wished she had stood up to her husband and defied him more often, but this was the era of the dutiful wife, and besides, she said, "You didn't argue with Paul Farmer, you just didn't." She also said, "We knew that he loved us."

In the turret, the Warden had constructed a tier of three bunks for the boys. P.J.'s was on top. He'd lie on it and read and do his homework while down below his brother Jeff practiced playing the drums, now and then declaring, "And this is the Krupa beat." P.J. excelled in school, regardless. He had some advantages, he'd say. The kind of father who thought it reasonable to house his family in a bus was also the kind who saw no reason P.J. shouldn't keep a large aquarium inside. Farmer insisted that he never really felt deprived throughout his childhood, though he did allow, "It *was* pretty strange." He remembered coming back to the campground on a school bus once and an African American classmate saying to him, "Is this where you stay at?" They remained at the campground for five years, and took trips away in the bus.

The Warden hadn't fully figured out the vehicle's wiring—he never did—and every time they pulled into a campground and plugged into a power outlet, there was a fifty-fifty chance that whoever did the plugging in would insert the plug wrong, reversing the polarity, and get a nasty shock. The boys would argue: "I did it last time!" The Warden seems not to have thought about labeling the plug, maybe because he didn't take a turn at inserting it himself. He was too busy at other tasks, Ginny would tell me with a smile. One time, returning from a trip to Massachusetts, his jury-rigged device for towing a car behind the bus malfunctioned, in a rainstorm on an interstate. The Blue Bird Inn slithered off the highway, then plunged down a steep embankment, then flipped onto its roof. The turret kept the bus from rolling. Miraculously, no one got seriously injured. But it took the Warden some months to repair, more or less, their living quarters.

When Farmer told me this story, I asked him where he'd stayed in the meantime.

"In a tent. Of *course*. What kind of a question is that?"

There were times inside the bus when the Warden would dance around and sing, times when he'd read them Shakespeare plays and books such as *Aesop's Fables*. But at least for Farmer's older sister, Katy, even his reading aloud could be nerve-racking. There was *The Swiss Family Robinson*. When he'd read a little way into that tale of a ship-wrecked family which finds happiness by living rustically on an island, Katy thought to herself, "Uh-oh." Later, when he got a few pages into *Robinson Crusoe*, she thought, "No! Please!" There had been other ominous signs. The Warden had never gone to sea, but even back in Alabama he'd been buying boating magazines. He had a great stack of them by now.

Around the time P.J. entered high school, the Warden bought at public auction an old Liberty launch, a fifty-foot-long empty hull with a hole in it, which he repaired. Then he took a year off from his paying jobs: he was teaching school and working with retarded adults in Brooksville. He built a cabin for the boat, cussing and fuming, learning his ship's carpentry, such as it was, as he went along. In the middle of his labors—the whole family had to pitch in—he started running short of cash, and he announced to P.J. and the two younger boys, "We're going to pick citrus."

P.J. said, "But, Dad, white people don't pick citrus."

"Yeah? I'll give you white people."

Most of the workers up on ladders in the orange trees were black, in fact. P.J. heard them talking from tree to tree in a strange language and asked his father what it was. "Creole. They're Haitians," the Warden explained. To young Paul, he described, briefly, the epic poverty of their country. But P.J. didn't get to know any Haitians then. The Farmers didn't work in the groves long enough. The pay was meager. After a few days, the Warden called it quits. He went back to work on the boat, which he named the *Lady Gin,* after his wife. When he declared it finished, he bought a generator for it and a fair amount of fishing gear that they really couldn't afford but that, he insisted, would pay for itself in no time. According to his plan, the boat would make them truly independent. It would serve as both their home and a source of revenue, through commercial fishing.

Their first voyage began on a calm and sunny day, the Warden at the helm. They steamed out into the Gulf of Mexico, far out of sight of land. They anchored in the shallow waters of the gulf, had lunch, and swam, P.J. and his siblings cavorting all around the boat. But they hauled up only a few edible fish, and then, that night, a storm blew in. The wind was howling, the boat was pitching at its anchor, and Ginny became terrified. Fear must have made her as implacable as her husband, because at some point that night, at her insistence, he tied a rope to the generator and threw it overboard as a second anchor. Meanwhile, down in their berths in the rocking, rolling cabin, the children were enjoying themselves immensely. "Cool, a storm." Years later Farmer's brother Jeff would tell me that he'd known all along his father was incompetent in boats. Even as they'd motored out that morning, he'd realized that the man knew nothing about navigation. "But the thing was—it was a strange feeling—you knew he didn't know what he was doing, but you also felt the security. That he would get us out of the situation. That nothing was really going to beat him." Ginny, for all the frights he put her through, would say of the Warden, "He was a great risk taker, and everything always turned out all right." She paused. "I mean, no one ever got seriously hurt."

The next day, heading landward, the Warden got lost and grazed a rock, but they made it safely into port. The *Lady Gin* went on a few other short, eventful voyages. On one of those, the Warden disregarded the channel markers—he seemed to think they represented arbitrary rules that he was not obliged to follow—and Jeff said, "Dad, you're not in the channel." The Warden said, "Shut up. What do you know about it?" and a moment later ran them hard aground. But for the most part, after its first and only fishing trip, the *Lady Gin* stayed moored in an otherwise uninhabited bayou on the Gulf Coast named Jenkins Creek.

On a bookcase shelf in his little house in the parched hills of inland

Haiti, Farmer kept a photograph of that other home. The *Lady Gin,* painted white but not very recently, floats moored to a metal pipe in the inlet. It's surrounded by marsh grasses, tall palm trees in the background. A gangplank leads to terra firma. A TV antenna sits on top of the cabin, and the cabin, a square superstructure planted on a rounded hull, doesn't quite fit. The Blue Bird Inn doesn't appear in the photograph, but it was parked nearby, ready for family excursions, on a dirt road beside the creek.

The Warden was happy there. He had his family where he seems to have wanted them—on an island, so to speak, safe from malign influences. As for young Paul, he loved the bayou, the starlit solitude, the osprey that lived in a nest off the *Lady Gin*'s starboard bow, the otters that would swim by, the alligators they'd hear barking at night. He'd save the money from his part-time jobs in Brooksville, at Hogan's Drugstore and at Biffburger, to buy materials for landscaping and for a fish pond across from their gangplank, and he does not seem to have been very discouraged by the high tides that periodically wiped out his handiwork.

The bayou life was hardest on Ginny. She worked all day at the Winn-Dixie and had to take care of six children and a husband on a boat. P.J.'s two brothers were growing up to be as large as their father. Their appetites were huge, and the refrigerator in the cabin was so small she had to restock it daily. When it rained, they put pots and pans beneath the leaks in the cabin's roof. At night cockroaches skittered in the bilge like a roomful of impatient women tapping their fingernails on tables. They washed their clothes in a Laundromat in town, and themselves and their dishes in the brackish water of the bayou. They got their drinking water some miles away, usually from a spigot outside a convenience store, surreptitiously filling the jugs that rattled around in the back of one or another of the vehicles that the Warden bought at auction—the Truck of Many Colors, or the olive drab army surplus sedan that they called the Staff Car, purchased by sealed bid for $288.

Once, on the lonesome road from Brooksville, the Staff Car overheated. They had no water with them, so the Warden ordered the boys to urinate into the radiator. The cars embarrassed P.J. and his siblings, especially the Staff Car. On the way to school one morning, they asked the Warden to drop them off a block away. Instead, he drove right into the bus lane in front of the whole school, honking the horn as he pulled up. "That'll show ya," he said.

Farmer would say of his childhood, "The way I tell myself the story is a little too neat. I'd like to be able to say that when I was young I lived in a trailer park, picked fruit with Haitians, got interested in migrant farmworkers, and went to Latin America. All true, but not the truth. We're asked to have tidy biographies that are coherent. Everyone does that. But the fact is, a perfectly discrepant version has the same ending."

Indeed, growing up without running water on a bus and a boat, with the Warden at the helm, hardly implies a single personality or fate. All Farmer's siblings grew up to live in houses. One of his sisters became a commercial artist, another the manager of community relations for a hospital's mental health programs, the third a motivational speaker. One brother was an electrician, and Jeff became a professional wrestler (known to his fans as Super J and to his family as the Gentle Giant).

No question, though, that Farmer's childhood was good preparation for a traveling life. Like all his siblings, he emerged from the bayou's waters with what he called a "very compliant GI system," and from dinners of hot dog–bean soup without much fussiness about food, and from years of cramped quarters with the ability to concentrate anywhere. He could sleep in a dentist's chair, as he did at night for most of one summer in a clinic in Haiti, and consider it an improvement over other places he had slept, and one might suppose that his fondness for a fine hotel and a good bottle of wine had the same origins. After the Staff Car, Farmer would say, it was hard to feel embarrassed or shy in front of anyone. He allowed that growing up as he did also probably relieved him of a homing instinct. "I never had a sense of a hometown. It was, 'This is my campground.' Then I got to the bottom of the barrel, and it was 'Oh, *this* is my hometown.' " He meant Cange.

It was partly to avoid the onerous houseboat chores assigned them by their father that Farmer and his siblings threw themselves into virtually every extracurricular activity that Hernando High in Brooksville offered. "No couch potatoes in the family," I said once to Farmer's mother. "No couch," she replied. Farmer was very popular in school, especially among the girls. The reason was simple, his mother said. "He listened to them." He was president of his senior class and went to Duke on a full scholarship.

To Farmer's great surprise, as Ginny remembered, he didn't get straight A's his first semester at college. Everything was new. He was soaking up high culture. He became drama critic and art critic for a student newspaper. The first play he'd ever seen was one he was sent to review. He was also discovering wealth. He met a fellow freshman in his dorm, named Todd McCormack, the son of a very successful sports agent. "How come you put your shirts in plastic?" Farmer asked, watching McCormack unpack. He was a brainy kid from a small south Florida town to whom hot showers were something of a novelty, who didn't have the right clothes or much spending money, and at Duke he had a couple of classmates whose father bought them a condominium so they wouldn't have to live in a dorm. For a time he dated a girl who kept her own horse near campus. Like about 60 percent of the student body, he joined a fraternity—and he became its social director. "I was pretty taken by it, by wealth," he remembered. "Nearly taken in."

There was a period, during his first two years at Duke, when to some of the family it seemed that P.J. might be making that customary American rite of passage and turning his back on them. He came home from college wearing a Lacoste shirt, and he said something to the effect that he couldn't wear clothes that weren't "preppy."

"Yeah, well," said the Warden, "Pel the preppy can still clean the bilge."

One time one of his younger sisters visited him at Duke, and over breakfast with P.J. and his current well-heeled girlfriend, his sister told in great graphic detail the story of how, in the bayou, she'd killed and disemboweled a pregnant water moccasin and made what she called a medusa hat for Paul out of the remains. The story had the effect she'd hoped for, the girlfriend pushing away her uneaten omelet while P.J. turned bright red trying to keep from laughing. Farmer remembered coming home from college once and the Warden opening the tailgate of his derelict pickup truck to reveal a chaos of worthless old lumber, a couple of wasps flying out, and the Warden saying, with his sardonic smile, "Someday, son, this will all be yours."

By then Farmer had quit his fraternity. He wrote them that he couldn't belong to an all-white organization. ("I received quite a frosty reply," he would say, in a tone of voice that implied this still surprised him.) He'd come to admire his father's distaste for putting on airs, and the man's fondness for underdogs—for the retarded adults he worked with and the neighbors at the trailer park who one year gave all the Farmer children piggy banks made out of old Clorox bottles—and his tendency to give money away to people who were truly poor. Farmer returned home less and less during his last years at Duke, but it wasn't as though he still intended, if he ever had, to trade in his old life for something fancier. "He had to get out from under his father," Ginny explained. "Back home everything would revert to the old order."

All the Farmer children, according to their mother, had craved their father's approval. He made it hard to get. Come home from high school with an A on a paper and he'd say, "Did anyone get an A plus?" The Warden loved sports. Farmer's brothers excelled at all. P.J. wasn't good at any. But he tried. It was an item of family lore that during the year he played baseball, the only thing he hit with a bat was the head of the coach's son, by accident. In high school, he went out for tennis and track, and would push himself so hard in races that he'd throw up at the finish lines. "When I think of it, I could just cry," Ginny would say. "He wanted to show his father he was an athlete, too, and his father would be so proud of him now." Actually, according to his brother Jeff, the Warden bragged about P.J. constantly—his test scores, his full scholarship to Duke—but only when P.J. wasn't around. "He was unbelievably proud of P.J., but he wouldn't tell him because he was the kind of guy who thought, I don't want your head to get too big."

In the Warden's evolving dream, his children grew up and had families and all settled down around him and Ginny in one large compound. Instead, one by one, they began leaving home. Then the man who owned the land beside Jenkins Creek died, the county purchased the property, and the Farmers had to leave. They moved ashore to a trailer home on two acres in a pine barren, off Star Road in Brooksville. Only the two youngest daughters, Jennifer and Peggy, were still around by then. They called their new home Star Road State Prison.

The *Lady Gin* had to be removed from its long anchorage. The Warden decided he would take it to a harbor farther south. He brought along only Jennifer, a teenager then. His navigation hadn't improved. His disdain for buoys and channel markers still endured. "He got the boat beached on a sandbar all night and couldn't get it off," Jennifer remembered. In the morning he told her, "We're just gonna burn it right here." He said he wanted to give their boat a "Viking funeral" out at sea. "No one else is going to live on it," he said. So he and Jennifer went through the boat and collected all the things they thought worth keeping, books and pictures mostly, and they loaded them into the dinghy—the *Mini Ginny*—which they rowed to a marina. They were in the process of buying gasoline for the Viking funeral when a man on the docks got wind of the Warden's mad intentions. "Don't do that. You'll kill yourselves. Besides, I want the engine." The man towed the *Lady Gin* off the sandbar and brought it into port. The Warden did burn the family boat, though, in a bonfire on land.

Looking back, Jennifer would say that her brother Paul and her father shared certain qualities. Above all, she thought, once they'd focused on a goal, neither one would quit. Her father had thought he could conquer the very elements. Nothing and no one ever seemed to intimidate him. "The only time I saw him vulnerable, *ever*, was that morning when he decided to burn the boat. Nothing was working right. The boat was aground, his kids were leaving, and he had no good helpers anymore."

He died a few years later, in July 1984, while playing a pickup game of basketball. He was forty-nine, and, to all outward appearances, had been a healthy man. He'd probably had a heart attack.

The telephone had not brought out the man's best qualities. When P.J. had learned he'd been accepted at Harvard Medical School, he'd called home from Haiti to tell his parents, and the Warden had said, "Oh yeah, we knew you'd get in." It had been, at moments anyway, a difficult relationship.

Farmer had a steady girlfriend by the time the Warden died. Not long after the funeral, she went to Florida with P.J. They stayed at Star Road State Prison. The Blue Bird Inn was parked there, semiderelict, and he went inside the bus and found some old books and letters. His girlfriend left on a brief errand. She remembered, "I came back and P.J. was sitting in the driver's seat, holding a letter his father wrote to him when he got into medical school. It said something like, 'I just want you to know how proud I am.' And P.J. was sobbing."

CHAPTER 6

Old college friends describe a boy who made friends easily, legions of them, at least as many female as male, and who had a "photographic memory" for facts about each one. "He'd ask about relatives that I didn't remember I'd even mentioned to him." If you went to lunch with him at a campus hangout, it could take half an hour to get to a table, he had to stop so often to chat with other people. He liked company when studying, and if you stayed up late with him to do it, you'd feel as though the work came more easily to him than to you, but then he'd start a food fight or make weird close-up images of his face on the copying machine, and later you'd all walk back across the silent campus loudly singing songs from *The Sound of Music*— "Raindrops on roses and whiskers on kittens."

After his first semester, Farmer started getting A's. He spent one summer and fall in Paris. He went there with only a little money and no job, and found a Franco-American family that wanted an au pair. His mother would send a five-dollar bill in her weekly letter, and he'd use it to go to plays. On his days off, he went to political demonstrations. "It's Saturday," the man of the house would say to him. "What demonstration did you go to today?" He took four courses in Paris, among them the last ever taught by the anthropologist Claude Lévi-Strauss, so infirm by then he had to be carried up onto the stage. By the time Farmer returned to Duke, he read, wrote, and spoke French fluently. He studied mostly science in his first two years of college, then focused on medical anthropology. He also read widely in subjects not assigned. Many professors were fond of him, and he of them. He wrote his senior honors thesis on "gender inequality and depression," no doubt in part because the medical anthropologists he knew were all psychiatrists. But he didn't claim any as a mentor. That distinction went to a German polymath named Rudolf Virchow, dead for the better part of a century.

Compared with other historical figures in medicine, such as Pasteur or Schweitzer or Florence Nightingale, Virchow isn't very well-known. Only one full-length biography of him exists. Yet he was, as one commentator writes, "the principal architect of the foundations of scientific medicine," the first to propose that the basic units of biological life were self-reproducing cells, and that the study of disease should focus on changes in the cell. Virchow made important contributions in oncology and parasitology, coined at least fifty medical terms still in use today, defined the pathophysiology of a host of diseases, including trichinosis, and led a successful campaign for compulsory meat inspection in Germany. He designed a sewage system for Berlin that transformed it from a fetid sty into one of Europe's healthiest cities. He founded a nursing school and hospitals. He was a practicing archaeologist and played an instrumental role in Heinrich Schliemann's excavations of Troy. He helped to define the field of medical anthropology. He was a physician and a teacher and a practicing politician, so nettlesome in opposition to Germany's imperial ambitions that Bismarck once challenged him to a duel.

Virchow published more than two thousand papers and dozens of books. At Duke, Farmer read some of his work in translation and several articles about him. Virchow's was a career to stir a brainy youth's imagination, an adventure that combined deeds and intellect, launched at an early age. When he was only twenty-six, the German government sent Virchow to Upper Silesia to report on an epidemic of what was then termed famine fever, now called relapsing fever. Virchow found a region impoverished by absentee landlordism, where the people, mainly Polish, lived principally on potatoes and vodka and suffered from endemic malaria and dysentery. In his report to the German government, he wrote that abysmal social conditions, which the government had fostered and done nothing to relieve, had caused the epidemic. This was forty years before medical science identified all the biological sources of relapsing fever—its vector is the louse—but subsequent discoveries would show that Virchow was right. Epidemics of the illness usually occur after social upheavals, in the ensuing overcrowding, poor hygiene, and malnutrition. In his report, Virchow expressed a fundamental law of epidemiology: "If disease is an expression of individual life under unfavorable conditions, then epidemics must be indicative of mass disturbances of mass life." His prescription for curing Upper Silesia was "full and unlimited democracy." This meant, among other things, establishing Polish as the official language, taxing the rich instead of the poor, getting the church out of the business of government, building roads, reopening orphanages, investing in agriculture. The government fired him. Virchow would write, "My politics were those of prophylaxis, my opponents preferred those of palliation."

He had a knack for aphorism. "Medicine is a social science, and politics is nothing but medicine on a large scale." "It is the curse of humanity that it learns to tolerate even the most horrible situations by habituation." "Medical education does not exist to provide students with a way of making a living, but to ensure the health of the community." "The physicians are the natural attorneys of the poor, and the social problems should largely be solved by them." This last was Farmer's favorite.

Virchow put the world together in a way that made sense to Farmer. "Virchow had a comprehensive vision," he said. "Pathology, social medicine, politics, anthropology. My model."

===

Farmer had acquired, partly through Virchow, a moral understanding of public health. While at Duke, he also found a subject.

He was reading very widely, in anthropology and history and sociology and political science. He was interested in current events, especially in the violent troubles in Latin America. In 1980, when Archbishop Oscar Romero was murdered by a right-wing death squad in El Salvador, faculty and students held a protest vigil at the Duke Chapel, and Farmer attended. He also did some reading about the branch of Catholicism called liberation theology, which Romero had been murdered for preaching. Latin American theologians had developed the doctrine, and in the late 1960s Latin America's Catholic bishops had endorsed some of its tenets. The bishop who had confirmed P.J. back in Brooksville had delivered a homily mainly about the perils of premarital sex. In the church documents Farmer read now, the Latin American bishops spoke about the oppression of the poor, calling it "institutionalized sin." They declared that the church had a duty to provide "a preferential option for the poor." Farmer remembered thinking, "Wow! This ain't the Catholicism I remember."

But he wasn't mainly impelled by politics or religion, he'd say. He felt more curious about the world than outraged. He had the sense that the truth about events in places like El Salvador lay hidden from most Americans. And it was in the same spirit mainly that he got interested in the migrant labor camps not far from Duke. "Here I am in the middle of a very affluent university, with a lot of comfortable ideas, and I met this nun. She was Belgian, Julianna DeWolf, working with the Friends of the United Farm Workers. And she was a fearless article. I just remember thinking she was much more radical and committed than anyone I'd met, arrogant and humble at the same time. The Haitian farmworkers thought the world of her." He met others like her—"church ladies," he called them—and he was impressed, not by their piety but by what they were willing to do on behalf of the migrant workers. "They were just so much more militant, if that's the word, than the WL's and academics. They were the ones standing up to the growers in their sensible nun shoes. They were the ones schlepping the workers to the clinics or court, translating for them, getting them groceries or driver's licenses."

In Sister Julianna's company, on tours of North Carolina tobacco plantations, he met a number of Haitians. The wretched conditions they lived in made the circumstances of his own childhood seem idyllic. He began reading everything he could find about Haiti. By the time he graduated, he knew enough to write an article of six thousand words about the Haitian farmworkers laboring in the fields near Duke. He called it "Haitians Without a Home." At home and abroad, he'd come to think, Haitians were the underdogs of underdogs, "the shafted of the shafted."

Farmer left Duke—he graduated summa cum laude—interested in all things Haitian. He visited Krome Detention Center in Florida and joined protests against what seemed to him the rank injustice of an American immigration policy that let in virtually every refugee from Cuba and sent nearly every fleeing Haitian back to hunger and disease and what had to be the Caribbean's cruelest, most self-serving dictatorship. By now he had certainly progressed, as he would put it, from curiosity to indignation. But curiosity remained.

The history of the country seemed worthy of a Homer or a Tolstoy or, especially to Farmer, a Tolkien. The landing of Columbus on the island that he named Hispaniola and the extermination of the Arawak Indians that followed. The division of the island between France and Spain, which left the French in possession of the island's western third, where they created an immensely lucrative and gruesome slave colony—a third of every new shipment of West African slaves died within three years. The slaves' long and bloody revolt, which began in 1791 and which not even Napoleon and forty thousand troops could put down. And at last, in 1804, the creation of Haiti, Latin America's first independent nation and the world's first black republic. But independence had been followed by nearly two hundred years of misrule, aided and abetted by foreign powers, especially France and the United States. (From 1915 to 1934, the U.S. Marines had occupied and run the country.)

To Farmer, Haiti's history seemed, indeed, like *The Lord of the Rings,* an ongoing story of a great and terrible struggle between the rich and the poor, between good and evil. What he read about the country's culture fascinated him. Haiti had its own music and literature. Paintings by Haitian artists hung in European and American museums. The people of Haiti had created their own complex religion, Voodoo— with a rather distant supreme deity and a host of other gods, a pantheon including Catholic saints. It was a system of belief that seemed all the more worth studying because it was so widely misunderstood and ridiculed. And the Haitian tongue, Creole, was not, as was sometimes said, "a coarse patois" but in essence a Romance language, derived from French and, in some of its phonetic habits and grammatical structures, also clearly African. It was unique to Haiti, lovely and expressive and born of grim necessity—the French masters had deliberately separated slaves who spoke the same languages, and the slaves had fashioned their own tongue. Farmer began to study Creole before he went to Haiti in the spring of 1983. He planned to spend about a year there.

He'd won a prize of one thousand dollars at Duke for an essay about Haitian artists, and he figured this should last him, since he'd read that the average Haitian lived on far less. He had worked as a volunteer in the emergency room at Duke's university hospital and had begun applying to the two schools, Harvard and Case Western Reserve, where one could get a joint degree as a doctor-anthropologist. He figured he'd find out if that was what he really wanted to become by trying out both disciplines in Haiti.

In 1983, when Farmer landed in Port-au-Prince, the airport was still named François Duvalier, in honor of the infamous Papa Doc, who had ruled the country, with liberal use of terror, from 1957 until his death in 1971. His reign was being continued now in the person of his son, Baby Doc—a little less crafty than his father but with the same proclivity for murdering political enemies and for stealing and misappropriating foreign aid. He would soon proclaim himself "president for life." In fact, the Duvaliers' three decades in power were nearly up, but no one knew that then. The Haiti that Farmer first encountered ranked as an exotic destination for tourists, including sex tourists—Haitians are a comely people, the majority desperately poor; one international guide for gay tourists reported in 1983, "Your partners will expect to be paid for their services but the charges are nominal." Port-au-Prince was a city full of slums, but it also had a few fancy neighborhoods and some good restaurants and hotels, and it was very safe for a tourist—patrolled by, among others, the Duvaliers' Praetorian guard, the men in dark glasses, the *tontons macoutes,* named for a mythical bogeyman, Uncle Sack, who stuffed bad children into his bag. They didn't harass tourists, not unless they looked in a suitcase and found a copy of Graham Greene's mordant, anti-Duvalierist novel of Haiti, *The Comedians*. Even then, they'd merely administer a harangue.

Farmer didn't bring his copy of the novel, and he didn't hang around in the city at first. During a brief postgraduate fellowship at the University of Pittsburgh, he had met a member of the Mellon family. They had used part of their fortune to build a hospital in Haiti, the Hôpital Albert Schweitzer, situated in the town of Deschapelles, in the lower Artibonite Valley. Farmer journeyed out there from Port-au-Prince almost as soon as he arrived. He had high expectations, and it was a good-looking hospital, he thought. But it was staffed mainly by white, expatriate doctors. He'd imagined something different—a hospital at least partly devoted to training Haitians to treat Haitians. Besides, the Schweitzer didn't have a job for him just then, in spite of his Mellon contact. He went back to the city, feeling, he'd say, "deflated."

He began looking around for other situations. He came across a small charity called Eye Care Haiti, with headquarters in Port-au-Prince. It conducted mobile "outreach clinics" in the countryside and kept a small house as a base for those operations out in the central plateau, in the town of Mirebalais. Farmer headed there.

CHAPTER 7

Years later Paul Farmer received this letter from a woman he wanted to marry:

Lovely Pel,

My inability to promise a life with you, as your wife, does not stem from a lack of love or deep, deep commitment to you. Indeed, as you probably know, I have not felt a serious ounce for anyone but you since 1983. My decision was based, instead, on trying to envision our life together and I saw us not matching (the only way we didn't fit). For a long time I thought I could live and work in Haiti, carving out a life with you, but now I understand that I can't. And that's simply not compatible with your life—the life you once told me you would like to lead even ten years ago. You pointed out to me once, during an emotional argument, that the qualities I love in you—that drew me to you—also cause me to resent you: namely your unswerving commitment to the poor, your limitless schedule and your massive compassion for others. You were right, and, as your wife, I would place my own emotional needs in the way of your important vision; a vision whose impact upon the poor (and the rest of us) can't be exaggerated . . .

I was lucky to meet you when I was young, young enough to feel as though I have always known you and lucky to have been hugely influenced and loved by you. In the end, I hope you know that as part of my histology you can never be replaced.

Her name was Ophelia Dahl. She came from Buckinghamshire in England. She had traveled to Haiti in January 1983, in order to please her father and with the intention, rather vague, of doing good works. She was eighteen—"a slightly mature eighteen," she would say—and was working as a volunteer for Eye Care Haiti. She was staying for a week at the Eye Care house in Mirebalais.

Back then Mirebalais was the country home of Madame Max Adolphe, formerly the warden of Fort Dimanche, where the Duvaliers sent their enemies, a prison likened by one historian to Buchenwald. Madame Max was now the national chief of the *tontons macoutes.* So Mirebalais was a place of some significance, different from most of the little towns scattered through the mountains and valleys farther north, in that it had intermittent electricity and radios playing at most hours, a small section of paved road at its center, ramshackle kiosklike stores beside the road, and a few places where you could buy a beer or a glass of the potent white rum called *clairin.* It also had a Teleco, a building near the center of town, where you could, with difficulty, get connected by phone to Port-au-Prince, or Brooklyn, or even Buckinghamshire.

Ophelia had wanted urgently to call home. A letter from her father had mentioned new troubles there, and she felt, irrationally and keenly, responsible for heading them off. She had gone into the Teleco, trying to think of the right things to say to her father. Her call didn't go through.

It was raining when she stepped outside, feeling glum. The rain had driven everyone else indoors. In fair weather, children would crowd around Ophelia, and people would call out *"Blan! Blan!"* as she passed—not intending rudeness, she had learned, but merely announcing the presence of an unusual sight. Here in the Haitian provinces, it was of course her white skin that made her stand out. But certainly she was a lovely young woman. In the midday heat of Haiti, her face would grow red blotches, but at normal temperature her skin had a lovely clarity.

Trudging moodily back to the Eye Care house in the warm rain, Ophelia looked up and, to her great surprise, saw a young white man standing on the building's balcony. "A pale and rangy fellow," she would remember. She'd been living among Haitians for months, eating their kind of food and beginning to speak their language, and she took some pride in the fact that she wasn't merely a tourist. She felt annoyed. Who was this *blan* on the balcony? What was he doing here on her turf? So she did what any well-bred English girl would do. She went inside and introduced herself to him.

The house had a common room with a cement floor, some wooden chairs, and a table. She and Paul sat down on either side of it and began to talk. Within minutes, she'd remember, she sensed that for the first time in months she didn't have to hold herself back, not even the part of herself that she thought of as "slightly outrageous," the part that liked bawdy humor and cussing. Before long she was telling this stranger about her aborted phone call and the hand-wringing feeling it left her with—trouble at home and she far away. She told him, "I want to write a nice letter to my father."

Paul smiled at her. "You should start with 'Dearest and indeed *only* Dad.'"

She laughed. At some point, Paul said, "Tell me about your family." Many years later a friend of hers would offer this recipe for seduction: "Go out to dinner and say, 'Tell me about your life.'" Ophelia would think of Paul and how, when he said those words, he made so many people feel he cared about only them at that moment. Of course, one knew that sometimes his interest was mixed with other motives, but he had this power because somehow one also knew that his interest was sincere. She told him about her movie star mother, Patricia Neal, and all the family tragedies—her mother's well-publicized cerebral hemorrhage and long convalescence, and currently well-publicized and angry breakup with Ophelia's father, the writer Roald Dahl. He was the one who had sent her to Haiti, in effect, by grousing that she should do something adventurous and useful. He worried that she lacked ambition. During her last two years of secondary school, she had studied geography, but before she'd boarded the plane to Port-au-Prince, she'd had to consult an atlas to find out where Haiti was.

She'd had a lot of pent-up thoughts and no one to tell them to, and now she did. Maybe any English-speaking stranger would have served the purpose, but this young man seemed close to ideal. She poured out her family's story, her sadness, her present worries, and Paul listened intently, never saying she shouldn't feel as she did, but only now and then suggesting ways she might accommodate her feelings. She was amazed. Here was this twenty-three-year-old American, who looked as though he was still molting adolescence, handsome enough but too pale and gangly and boyish-looking to be called dishy, and she thought, "How does *he* know what to say to me that would be comforting?"

She liked the way Paul responded to her near-celebrity. She didn't sense he was thinking, "I'm talking to a movie star's daughter!" He just seemed amused by the circumstance. He told her a little about his own family, and a few of the stories of his childhood, and these made her laugh. She gathered that he had come out to Mirebalais to see if he wanted to join up with Eye Care. So she described the various personalities on the team. She wouldn't have liked him half so much if he hadn't said, "Thank you for telling me that," with such evident feeling, with his eyes opened wide.

They talked until about three in the morning. For the next few days he went out with the team in its Land Rover. He had told her that he was in Haiti mainly to do anthropology. She wasn't quite sure what that meant. He had a tape recorder and a camera and a notebook, and, seated beside him, she watched him do his own watching from the truck. As they bumped along the dusty roads, past the miserable peasant huts, she asked him questions. Why were so many people sick? Why weren't the roads better? He would answer her, but warily at first, as if he was waiting to be sure just who she was. He was embarrassingly enthusiastic, though. When people by the roadside called out, *"Blan! Blan!"* he would call back, "Hi!" and grin and make floppy-wristed waves. Once you were no longer a tourist, you didn't *wave,* she thought. "Waving at your brown brothers?" she said.

Farmer turned to her. "What's that supposed to mean?"

He was trying to smile. Looking at him, she thought, "He's innocent about meanness." He was the sort of person who didn't feel compelled to tell you all his thoughts, but she sensed that if he did tell you some, if he let you in, and you made fun of him, it would be a long time before he'd open up again. For the first time in months she was in the company of someone she could have fun with, and she'd blown it. "I'm sorry, I'm sorry," she said. "I didn't mean it."

He smiled at her, and the next time someone called *"Blan!"* he waved just as before. She felt forgiven. He did other nerdy things, like telling her the Latin names of trees and shrubs. He wasn't shy at all. He seemed able to talk to anyone but was clearly most interested in talking to peasants—who were, he explained, the vast majority of Haitians, even in the urban slums. He took photographs. He made notes about the hospitals they visited. He asked peasants many questions. Where did they get their drinking water? What did they think caused illnesses? He recorded the conversations and transcribed them at night back at the Eye Care house. He was mastering Creole with enviable speed. She'd been in Haiti for months, and he had only recently arrived, yet by the end of their week of travel, he had surpassed her. He could almost, in the Haitian phrase, speak Creole like a rat.

At the end of that week in the countryside, the Eye Care team headed back toward Port-au-Prince. She and Paul sat together in the backseat on the long drive. By now, he was calling her by the nickname her family had given her, Min. He was regaling her with the myriad nicknames in his own family as they neared the steep, narrow part of National Highway 3 that scales down Morne Kabrit, Goat Mountain, toward the Cul-de-Sac Plain. The Rover began turning a corner beside the cliff, and they were thrown to one side together, and then up ahead they saw a carpet of mangoes spread across the road. Children dashed around, gathering up the fruit. A little farther on, a small, battered pickup truck lay on its side. Obviously, the tap-tap had been top-heavy with passengers and fruit, heading for market. Obviously, it had exhausted shock absorbers and bad brakes. Overturned baskets and mangoes were strewn all around. The passengers were market women, in head wraps, some sitting by the road looking dazed, others standing around talking heatedly. One woman lay near the truck, her body surrounded by mangoes and only partly covered with a piece of cardboard. There was a policeman at the scene. He told them cheerfully, three gold-framed teeth gleaming, that, yes, the woman had died. There was nothing to be done.

For Ophelia the scene behind them would become a fixture in her memories, like her first scent of Haiti—the acidic, garbagey smell that had hit her when she'd first arrived at the François Duvalier Airport. She looked over at Paul as they drove on toward the city. He was staring out the window. He had become, she would remember, "very, very silent."

They didn't become lovers that spring, but they saw each other almost every day over the next month or so, sometimes on Eye Care's outreach expeditions, more often in Port-au-Prince. When they were both in the city, she would walk over to his place after work. He lived in an old ruin of a mansion, covered with balconies and wooden fretwork, set in a garbage-strewn lot. It belonged to an art dealer. The wife of a previous owner—so the story went—had gone into labor one night during a period when Baby Doc had imposed a curfew on the city, and the husband had run out to get help and been shot dead on the street. The house was huge and empty, except for Paul and one other tenant, a Haitian woman, who would sometimes cook meals out in the courtyard, the smell of burning charcoal rising into Paul's windows. His room was on the second floor. It had many windows with old, elaborate wooden shutters opening onto balconies. Through the windows you could see a large part of the city and the waterfront and, off to one side, the tents and cardboard huts in a slum called La Saline.

She often found him up in his room writing. He had composed a poem, called "The Mango Lady," dedicated "To Ophelia." He read it aloud. The third verse began:

> We start, eyes drawn reluctantly back
> over baskets, to the dead mango lady
> stretched stiff on her bier of tropical fruit.
> She is almost covered by a cardboard strip,
> like the flag of her corrugated country,
> a flimsy strip too thin to hide the wounds.

No doubt being far from home simplified their courtship, so that it didn't even seem like one. When they went out, she paid the way. She had money. He didn't have much. It seemed only sensible and natural that she share hers. And he shared his superior knowledge of Haiti. He told her about Madame Max, for instance—teasing her, explaining that the Eye Care house sat on Madame Max's land, so that, in effect, Ophelia was working for the *tontons macoutes*. One time she said to him, "I met this interesting guy at the Oloffson. He says he's the model for Petit Pierre in Graham Greene's book *The Comedians*." Paul explained that this was true, and that the clownish little man she'd met was a Duvalierist informant. Paul was educating her, she felt, though not deliberately. Usually, she asked the questions. Often, a little artfulness was needed. If he made a cryptic or broad statement, it was best not to challenge him, because then he might grow reticent. Better to say, "Tell me more." Up in his room in the haunted house, she initiated many talks—"our long, windy discussions," she'd say years later.

"What is anthropology exactly?"

He told her, in effect—I am using words he would put in print in an article about a year and a half later—that anthropology concerned itself less with measurement than with meaning. As in mastering a language, one had to learn not just the literal meanings of words but also their connotations, and to grasp those one had to know the politics and economic systems and histories of a place. Only then could you really understand an event like the mango lady's death.

In the article he wrote the following year, Farmer would use phrases such as "highly reticulated relations among disease, nutritional status, socioeconomic factors, and health and illness beliefs and practices." As a rule, he didn't speak much more plainly about subjects like the mango lady, but Ophelia made her own translations. Accidents happen. Sure. But not every bad thing that happens is an accident. There was nothing accidental about the wretchedness of the road down Morne Kabrit or the overloaded tap-tap, or the desperation of a peasant woman who had to get to market and make a sale because otherwise her family would go hungry. These circumstances all had causes, and the nearest ones were the continuing misrule of the Duvaliers and the long-standing American habit of lavishing aid on dictators such as Baby Doc, who used the money to keep himself and the Haitian elite in luxury and power and spent almost nothing on things like roads and transportation.

Before she'd met Paul, Haiti had seemed merely vivid—terrible and strange. The worm a full foot long that she'd seen wriggling out of a baby's anus in the hospital where she first worked. The numberless children with diarrheal diseases. The daily national anthem ceremony in front of the presidential palace, where by decree everyone had to stop and face the tinny music or suffer the wrath of the *macoutes*. Now she had someone to translate Haiti to her. In the process Paul laid out a comprehensive theory of poverty, of a world designed by the elites of all nations to serve their own ends, the pieces of the design enshrined in ideologies, which erased the histories of how things came to be as they were. And he knew the details for Haiti, a catastrophe covered with the fingerprints of the Western powers, most of all those of France and the United States.

Ophelia gazed out the windows of Paul's room in the mansion as he read his latest poem to her. Poverty was his subject, she thought, and the windows of this haunted house were his observation post. He was looking for a better one. His plans weren't clear, but his aims seemed to be. He'd come here to do ethnography, the kind of anthropology he most admired—learning about a culture, not through books and artifacts but from the people who had inherited and were making culture. His special field was going to be medical ethnography. He wanted to learn everything about morbidity and mortality in the most disease-ridden country in the hemisphere. He'd write about what he discovered and in this way, he told her, "lend a voice to the voiceless." He'd also be a doctor. He wasn't sure which branch of medicine he'd choose. Maybe psychiatry. In any case, he'd be a doctor to poor people. Maybe he'd end up working in Africa or an American inner city.

Drawing him out, Ophelia felt both enthralled and disturbed. During one of their long talks in his room, she found herself thinking, "Oh dear, oh good, my life has changed." Years later she would tell me, "I think there's a point where you realize the world has just been revealed to you. It's like realizing your parents are both good and bad. It's sort of, Oh no, things will never be quite the same again."

She was, after all, very young. A person five years older could be a credible mentor, though now and then he'd say something that reminded her he wasn't very old himself. Before she left Haiti, late that spring, she told him she was going home to do premedical studies. She was going to become a doctor, too.

"Good," he said earnestly. He had finished his own premed work. "You know what you should do? Make flash cards."

They promised to write.

===

Paul had asked Ophelia to call his parents when she got home, but he had neglected to tell her that the Warden, still very much alive in 1983, had a rule that his daughters call home every night before they drove back to Star Road State Prison from their after-school jobs in Brooksville. And Farmer also hadn't told her that his sister Peggy had lately affected a convincing English accent.

She made the call. "Hello, Mr. Farmer. My name's Ophelia and I just came from Haiti. I was just with Paul and he sends his love, and he wants you to know he's all right."

"Yeah, yeah, yeah. All right, Peggy, knock it off."

"No, my name is *Ophelia* and I was just with Paul."

"I'll *feel ya,* Peggy. Get on home!" said the Warden and hung up.

Ophelia called back and managed to convince him eventually. The Warden apologized. She could hear laughter in the background.

Ophelia had left Paul several contemporary novels. By the time she got back to England, a letter had arrived, a book report of sorts. "The entire novel is more fun if you've read Dante's *Inferno,* Joyce's *Ulysses* (the chapter in which Bloom brings Molly breakfast in bed), Homer, Proust (*À la Recherche du Temps Perdu*), and *The Maids,* a play by Genet." At the end, he had written, "P.S.: You're a slut for leaving me here alone." Increasingly ardent requests for a letter followed: "You trollop you. Why haven't you dispatched any passenger pigeons in my direction?" If she didn't write *"tout de suite,"* he'd lock her in a broom closet with a rather unattractive mutual acquaintance of theirs, give both of them "potent aphrodisiacs," and "take away the Lavoris." For a time, she didn't write him back. She wasn't sure why. Maybe she was just being lazy. She still intended to become a doctor, and she hated to think that she might never see him again.

Soon after she got back to Europe, her father took her to lunch with Graham Greene, who Paul had said was one of his favorite writers. The elderly novelist, tall and stooped, seemed genuinely glad for news of Haiti, especially of the egregious Petit Pierre. He inscribed her copy of *The Comedians,* "To Ophelia, who knows the real Haiti." If he really thought that of her, she wondered, what would he have made of Paul Farmer?

CHAPTER 8

It was soon after Ophelia left that Farmer first saw Cange, in late May 1983. Still searching for a place to do his work, he had traveled back to the central plateau and was spending some time in the company of a Haitian Anglican priest named Fritz Lafontant. He was a small but imposing man, with a grand, almost leonine countenance and a forceful manner, sometimes abrupt. With assistance from the Episcopal Diocese of Upper South Carolina, Lafontant administered a rather rudimentary one-doctor health clinic in Mirebalais. He and his wife had also helped to build schools and to organize community councils and women's groups and programs for adult literacy in several small, impoverished towns in the region. Cange was one of those. Lafontant had arranged and supervised the construction of a chapel and the beginnings of a school in Cange. Farmer rode out there from Mirebalais in the back of the priest's pickup truck.

Spring in Haiti is usually a fairly wet season, and much of the route was green, especially the stretch along the Artibonite where the river had cut a gorge too steep for agriculture. Farmer remembered admiring the trees and foliage there and the rushing river. Then the large dam and the reservoir heaved into view, and after that he found himself staring through clouds of grayish dust—dust in his hair, dust up his nose, dust adhering to his sweaty skin—at an utterly changed landscape, with scarcely any trees, colored in shades of brown and white, a landscape he would remember as "amazingly, biblically, dry and barren." Cange, the squatter settlement, lay in the midst of this arid desolation, half a mile up the road from the huge freshwater reservoir.

Most of the dwellings were crude wooden lean-tos with dirt floors, constructed, it seemed, without much conviction, as a friend of his would later put it. Farmer noticed especially the roofs of these tiny hovels, roofs made of banana-bark thatch, patched with rags, clearly leaky. Back in Mirebalais the roofs of rusty, thin metal, of "tin," had seemed to him like the emblems of poverty. "But," he would say, "the absence of tin, in Cange, screamed, 'Misery.'" Most of the adults he saw and talked to were clearly dejected. It was as if, he thought, the people who had built these miserable lean-tos weren't convinced that they'd ever live in anything better, indeed expected things to get worse. Many, perhaps the majority, were obviously ill, and there was no medicine of any sort being provided there. They seemed like the people he'd seen in waiting rooms in the dreadful public clinics he'd visited. It was as if the whole makeshift settlement were one of those waiting rooms. Haiti had already redefined poverty for him. Cange redefined it again. An individual might exist in misery this great almost anywhere, but it was hard to imagine an entire community poorer and sicker than this.

Père Lafontant's party spent the night in Cange, on the floor of the school's classrooms, sleeping on old army blankets. Farmer remembered waking up at 2:00 A.M. to go to the bathroom and pissing loudly in a bucket, a sound he recalled from his days on the bus, preferable to stepping outside in the night, among the parts of creation that had always given him the creeps—huge bugs and, especially, tarantulas.

=

He didn't stop in Cange for long, not on that first visit. He kept traveling around Haiti, hitching rides from *blan* sometimes, sometimes riding in tap-taps among the peasants and their chickens and their baskets full of mangoes. He came down with dysentery, probably because his budget obliged him to eat food sold on the streets of the cities and towns. He remembered lying in a grubby hospital in Port-au-Prince, on a floor that lacked a toilet, and a middle-aged American woman, a public health expert whom he'd gotten to know, visiting him there. She was saying that, if he got any sicker, she was going to take him back to the States, and he was telling her, No, no, he was all right, while thinking, Please take me home. When he recovered, he went on sampling Haiti, and anthropology and medicine in the context of Haiti. He attended Voodoo ceremonies, talked to peasants about their lives, and found his way, among other places, to a hospital in Léogâne, a town about twelve miles west of Port-au-Prince, on Haiti's southern peninsula. He worked there for a while as a volunteer, assisting the nurses and doctors.

Farmer told me that he found his life's work not in books or in theories but mainly through experiencing Haiti. "I would read stuff from scholarly texts and know they were wrong. Living in Haiti, I realized that a minor error in one setting of power and privilege could have an enormous impact on the poor in another." The eradication of the Creole pig, or the dam at Péligre, for example.

He was already attracted to liberation theology. "A powerful rebuke to the hiding away of poverty," he called it. "A rebuke that transcends scholarly analysis." In Haiti, the essence of the doctrine came alive for him. Almost all the peasants he was meeting shared a belief that seemed like a distillation of liberation theology: "Everybody else hates us," they'd tell him, "but God loves the poor more. And our cause is just." The Marxists Farmer had read, and many of the intellectuals he knew, disdained religion, and it was true that some versions of Christianity, and more than a few missionaries, invited impoverished Haitians into what Père Lafontant called "the cult of resignation," into accepting their lot patiently, anticipating the afterlife. But the Christianity of the peasants Farmer talked to had a different flavor: "the shared conviction that the rest of the world was wrong for screwing them over, and that someone, someone just and perhaps even omniscient, was keeping score." He felt drawn back toward Catholicism now, not by his own belief but in sympathy with theirs, as an act of what he'd call "solidarity." He told me, "It was really the experience of seeing people up there in Cange, or in some awful hospital, or at a funeral, or knowing that people were awaking in their huts to two rooms full of hungry kids *and still going on.* Religion was the one thing they still had."

How could a just God permit great misery? The Haitian peasants answered with a proverb: *"Bondye konn bay, men li pa konn separe,"* in literal translation, "God gives but doesn't share." This meant, as Farmer would later explain it, "God gives us humans everything we need to flourish, but he's not the one who's supposed to divvy up the loot. That charge was laid upon us." Liberation theologians had a similar answer: "You want to see where Christ crucified abides today? Go to where the poor are suffering and fighting back, and that's where He is." Liberation theology, with its emphasis on the horrors of poverty and on redressing them in the here and now, its emphasis on service and remediation, seemed to fit the circumstances of Haiti. And it suited Farmer temperamentally because, for all his scholarship and interest in theories, his strongest impulses were pragmatic. He only seemed like a nerd. He would tell me years later, with undeniable accuracy, "I'm an action kind of guy."

Looking back at this first year of living in Haiti, Farmer would speak of the feeling that many things in his mind coalesced into a vision of his life's proper work. But, he'd insist, this happened in stages, not all at once. "For me, it was a process, not an event. A slow awakening as opposed to an epiphany." Then he remembered an incident from the time he spent in Léogâne. Repossessing it, he said that perhaps there had been an epiphany after all.

Working as a medical volunteer at the Hôpital St. Croix in Léogâne, he got to know a young American doctor. "He loved the Haitians," Farmer said. "He was a very thoughtful guy." The man had worked in Haiti for about a year. Now, in a few days, he was going back to the United States. "I realized, hearing him talk, that something had happened to me already," Farmer said. "I wasn't feeling judgmental. Haiti was something he was seeing that he could leave and erase from his mind, and I was thinking, Could I do that? He was leaving Haiti, really leaving in body and mind, and I realized I was going to have trouble with that."

"Isn't it going to be hard to leave?" he asked the young doctor.

"Are you kidding? I can't wait. There's no electricity here. It's just brutal here."

"But aren't you worried about not being able to forget all this? There's so much disease here."

"No," the doctor said. "I'm an American, and I'm going home."

"Right. Me, too," said Farmer.

He thought about that conversation all the rest of the day and into the evening. "What does that mean, 'I'm an American'? How do people classify themselves?" He understood the doctor's position, but he didn't really know his own. The only thing he knew for sure was that he would become a doctor himself.

Later on that night, a young woman arrived at the hospital, pregnant and in the throes of malaria. "She had a very high parasitemia," Farmer remembered. "Bad malaria. She went into a coma, and you know—I didn't know the details then, I do now because it's my specialty—she needed a transfusion, and her sister was there. So there was no blood and the doctor told her sister to go to Port-au-Prince to get her some blood, but he said that she would need money. I had no money. I ran around the hospital, and I rounded up fifteen dollars. I gave her the money and she went away, but then she came back and she didn't have enough for both a tap-tap and the blood. So meanwhile the patient started having respiratory distress and this pink stuff started coming out of her mouth. The nurses were saying, 'It's hopeless,' and other people were saying, 'We should do a cesarean delivery.' I said, 'There's got to be some way to get her some blood.' Her sister was beside herself. She was sobbing and crying. The woman had *five kids*. The sister said, 'This is terrible. You can't even get a blood transfusion if you're poor.' And she said, 'We're all human beings.' "

The words—*tout moun se moun*—seemed like the answer to the question he'd asked himself earlier that day. Was being an American a sufficient identity unto itself? "She said that again and again," he remembered. "We're all human beings."

The woman and her unborn baby died. Afterward, the sister lavished thanks on Farmer. And of course this made him feel more acutely his failure at emergency fund-raising. He was obviously upset, and the doctors and nurses seemed to focus their attention on him. The nurses were saying, "Poor Paul. What a sweet young man." And he knew what the doctors were thinking: "He's new here, he's green, he's naïve." Remembering this years later, he was still framing his retort: "Yeah, but I got staying power. That's the thing. I wasn't naïve, in fact."

Or perhaps he was, a little. He decided to raise money to buy the hospital its own blood-banking equipment. He wrote to his relatives and the parents of his friends from Duke. He was seeing dreadful things in Haiti, he wrote. He described the project. Many checks arrived. In the end, he collected a few thousand dollars. He was elated. He wrote to Ophelia, "I'm off to Léogâne for a meeting with the director of Hôpital St. Croix to discuss BIG PLANS." But not long afterward, Ophelia received another letter: "My stint down here at the hospital isn't turning out exactly as I thought it would. It's not that I'm unhappy working here. The biggest problem is that the hospital is not for the poor. I'm taken aback. I really am. Everything has to be paid for in advance."

The central imperative of liberation theology—to provide a preferential option for the poor—seemed like a worthy life's goal to him. Of course, one could pursue it almost anywhere, but clearly the doctrine implied making choices among degrees of poverty. It would make sense to provide medicine in the places that needed it most, and there was no place needier than Haiti, at least in the Western Hemisphere, and he hadn't seen any place in Haiti needier than Cange. He didn't stick around in Léogâne to see the blood bank get installed. He'd found out that the hospital would charge patients for its use. He told me he had these thoughts, as he headed back toward the central plateau: "I'm going to build my own fucking hospital. And there'll be none of that there, thank you."

≡

When he returned from Léogâne to the central plateau, Farmer went to work for a while at Père Lafontant's clinic in Mirebalais. It resembled a lot of the clinics he'd seen in his months of exploring Haiti. Patients waited in a line for a visit with the lone doctor, who didn't bother to get their medical histories or give them real physical exams. "A perfunctory exchange with a doctor who'd rather have been any-where else but there," Farmer would remember. "Then the patients took their filthy corncob-stoppered bottles to the 'pharmacy' and *paid* to have them glug-glug filled up, with cough medicine and vitamins. A sorry spectacle, which included, at times, the staff yelling at the pa-tients for bringing really, *really* filthy bottles."

With Père Lafontant's blessing, Farmer began to focus on the wretched, dusty squatter settlement up the road in Cange. It was a big moment in his life. "Going up to Cange, which was back then a truly awful place compared to Mirebalais, was for me, bizarrely, a relief. *No clinic at all was a relief!* Not because there wasn't an urgent need for a clinic in Cange. I just knew I couldn't work in a clinic like that one in Mirebalais, which was, I had learned, altogether representative of other clinics for poor Haitians. And I also knew, I hope, that it wasn't about how I felt or how the hapless Haitian doctor felt. It was about the patients and their awful outcomes."

Cange needed a clinic, a hospital, a community health system. In Farmer's conception, the facilities should provide services to the des-titute for free, and those services should meet the real needs of the place and of individual patients. So the first step was to find out exactly what the needs were. Farmer began modestly, with a preliminary health census. He enlisted five Haitians, all about his age, all of whom had gone at least as far in school as the first year of junior high, and they went from hut to hut through Cange and two neighboring villages, tallying up the numbers of families, recent births and deaths, and the apparent causes of morbidity and mortality. That first survey was rather informal, but it confirmed what Farmer had already sus-pected. Mortality among infants and juveniles was "horrific." He learned, too, about the central importance of "maternal mortality"—how the deaths of mothers, common events in those squatter settle-ments, led to skeins of catastrophes in families, to hunger and prostitution, to disease and other deaths.

This first survey was just a small beginning, a piece of an apprenticeship in public health and medicine and also anthropology. In Cange in early 1984, Farmer had another memorable encounter with malaria, in its way as instructive as the one back in Léogâne. The patient was a young woman. Her father decided to have her treated by a local *houngan,* a Voodoo priest, but after a lot of discussion, the mother agreed to let Farmer and a Haitian doctor treat her with chloroquine as well. She recovered. In an essay which he titled "The Anthropologist Within," Farmer wrote that, in the aftermath of that case, he'd wondered obsessively about the role anthropology should assume in his life. He'd been taught that an ethnographer should observe, not try to change what was being observed. But practiced in that way, anthropology seemed "impotent" in the face of "everyday problems of adequate nutrition, clean water, and illness prevention." It's clear by the end of the essay that anthropology now interested him less as a discipline unto itself than as a tool for what he called "intervention." He had settled not for a synthesis between observing and acting, but for doctoring and public health work that would be partly guided by anthropology.

Its uses were obvious. A doctor who knew nothing about local beliefs might end up at war with Voodoo priests, but a doctor-anthropologist who understood those beliefs could find ways to make Voodoo *houngans* his allies. A doctor who didn't understand local culture would probably mistake many patients' complaints for bizarre superstitions, or at best be utterly baffled—by the female complaint called *move san, lèt gate,* for instance. The condition was said to be brought on by *sezisman,* that is, by a surprise or by someone's frightening action. *Move san,* "bad blood," could follow, and produce in turn *lèt gate,* a condition in which a nursing mother's milk was spoiled or stopped flowing. None of this would be mysterious to a young ethnographer-doctor who, like Farmer, was willing to puzzle out the social meanings of the syndrome. Farmer would write, "The most striking thing about *move san* disorder is the lurid extremity of its symbolism: two of the body's most vital constituents, blood and milk, are turned to poisons. The powerful metaphors serve, it may be inferred, as a warning against the abuse of women, especially pregnant or nursing ones."

In the course of his research on *move san, lèt gate,* he consulted a local Haitian woman, asking her about the herbal remedies for the condition. She gave him the information and then told him, in effect, "Surely you are collecting these leaves in order to better understand their power and improve their efficacy." This was a lesson reiterated. The people of Cange weren't interested in having their suffering merely scrutinized; he should be interested in both research and action.

Farmer was probably fortunate—certainly he thought so—to have done some work in anthropology and medicine and public health in Haiti before he studied those disciplines at Harvard. He had a gift for academic pursuits, but Haiti ensured that his taste for them would be limited.

=

Farmer entered Harvard Medical School in the fall of 1984. He was only twenty-four. Then again, he told me once, "I was fully formed at twenty-three." He meant, I think, that by then he had his philosophy and worldview in order, and knew that he wanted to marry them to action, first of all in Cange. He didn't linger in Cambridge. He stayed around Harvard just long enough to get oriented and to gather up textbooks, which he took with him back to the central plateau.

At the medical school, the first two years of the curriculum consisted mainly of large lecture courses. Often, Farmer would show up in Cambridge just in time for lab practicums or exams. Then he'd go back to Haiti. It wasn't as though no one noticed. By the second year, his classmates had nicknamed him Paul Foreigner. But while this kind of commuting by a student was almost certainly unprecedented, it would have been hard for any professor to disapprove. The young man was trying to bring medicine to people without doctors. Besides, his grades were excellent, some of the best in his class.

CHAPTER 9

The combination of Harvard and Haiti had begun to form a new kind of belief in Farmer. He would tell me years later: "The fact that any sort of religious faith was so disdained at Harvard and so important to the poor—not just in Haiti but elsewhere, too—made me even more convinced that faith must be something good."

And if the landless peasants of Cange needed to believe that someone omniscient was keeping score, by now Farmer felt the need to believe something like that himself. In the peasant phrase, an unnecessary death was "a stupid death," and he was seeing a lot of those. "Surely someone is witnessing this horror show?" he'd say to himself. "I know it sounds shallow, the opiate thing, needing to believe, palliating pain, but it didn't feel shallow. It was more profound than other sentiments I'd known, and I was taken with the idea that in an ostensibly godless world that worshiped money and power or, more seductively, a sense of personal efficacy and advancement, like at Duke and Harvard, there was still a place to look for God, and that was in the suffering of the poor. You want to talk crucifixion? I'll show you crucifixion, you bastards."

When Ophelia went back to the central plateau to work with Paul, in the summer of 1985, she saw that, when he dressed up now in Haiti, he often wore a large wooden cross hanging outside his shirt. But the apparatus only reinforced a quality of "priestliness" that she'd sensed in him before, and that quality was far from thorough. He would say, some years later, that he had "faith," then add, "I also have faith in penicillin, rifampin, isoniazid, and the good absorption of the fluoroquinolones, in bench science, clinical trials, scientific progress, that HIV is the cause of every case of AIDS, that the rich oppress the poor, that wealth is flowing in the wrong direction, that this will cause more epidemics and kill millions. I have faith that those things are true, too. So if I had to choose between lib theo, or any ology, I would go with science as long as service to the poor went along with it. But I don't have to make that choice, do I?"

He'd never cared much about the religious dogma he'd been taught as a child, and he didn't believe in most of it now. He would say, for instance, "I'm still looking for something in the sacred texts that says, 'Thou shalt not use condoms.' " He was still the very young man who would challenge Ophelia to mango-eating contests that turned into slimy food fights, and he was quite willing to ignore the injunctions about chastity that the bishop had uttered at his confirmation in Florida years ago. Indeed, he was happy to skip church services in order to violate those injunctions. Ophelia remembered the afternoon when she "gave" herself to him—she chuckled at the term. It was a Sunday. They were in Mirebalais and got caught in a rainstorm, and ran back to Père Lafontant's rectory. The building was empty because everyone else was in church, and in Haiti church services tend to last a long time. Moreover, most Haitians don't like being out in the rain. "You knew that, until it ended, no one would be coming," she said. "We took a shower together." She remembered the sound of the rain on the roof, the smell of the smoke from the fire out in the courtyard lit for Sunday dinner. The moment, she said, still stood in her memory as the most romantic of her life.

She spent the whole summer in Haiti with Paul. In the evenings, over coffee, she'd help him with his formal medical education. She'd try to help, that is. He had distilled the contents of his medical texts onto index cards. He had great piles of them, thousands of flash cards. On one side he'd have written, in an elegant, left-handed script, a question such as "What's gout got to do with lysosomes?" and he'd have added the symbols for musical notes around the words, indicating that the question should be sung. The question side of a card might read, for example, "Show me, sir, the lesions in Horner's syndrome, & oculomotor nerve paralysis. And what the divvil's an Argyll Robertson pupil?" The answers on the back often included drawings—many of them lovely, Ophelia thought—in that case a drawing of the neural pathways of the eye.

Ophelia looked through the stack of index cards for a question that Paul might answer wrong, hoping he would. It felt good to be able to read him the correct answer, as if she was actually helping. "Okay, P.J., what's dystrophic calcification?"

"When abnormal deposition of calcium salts takes place in necrotic tissues, it's known as dystrophic calcification." He'd lift a finger in the air. "Of course, it's *not* caused by hypercalcemia." He'd smile. "Metastatic calcification *is* associated with hypercalcemia, however."

She'd stare at the back of the index card, trying not to look let down. "Right! Very good, P.J."

They walked to villages from time to time. On the way he'd point out plants. "Indigo," he'd say, and then with an eager smile, "What's the Latin name?"

He'd been doing this since she'd first met him. At moments, she wondered if he was trying to make her feel uneducated. "No, you twit, of course not," she thought. "He just likes to say the names. It's one of his ideas of fun."

But it was hard to avoid comparing herself with him. At almost every hut they visited, food would appear, a great deal of it unsavory to both of them—items from what Paul called "the fifth food group"—and, making faces at each other when their hosts weren't looking, they pretended to munch happily on things like meat-filled pastries that smelled like sweat. Then one time their hosts presented each of them with what looked like a fried egg afloat in pig fat and gristle, and she took a bite and almost gagged on it. When the hosts turned away for a moment, she handed her plate to Paul, whispering, "Here, you eat it." He took the plate and slurped the contents down. Then he looked at her and smiled. "B minus," he said. On the way back they laughed about the incident, and yet of all the times she'd eaten things that she could hardly bear to look at, this one occasion when she failed the test stood out for her.

Coming down a steep trail in one of the hills around Cange, she lost her footing momentarily. There were Haitians nearby. "Watch your step!" someone called to her in Creole. She felt the muscles in her jaw flex. Did they think she was a weakling? An elderly man came up to her and offered her his walking stick. "No, I'm fine!" she said. Paul's face looked stern. "Don't refuse something like that," he said to her emphatically. "It's an incredible gift." Of course he was right. Her cheeks burned.

They slept in different quarters in Cange—the patriarch of the place was, after all, a priest. One night, about to turn in, she decided that tomorrow she'd get up earlier than Paul. She set her alarm clock for five. She woke to the sound of his voice, singing up to her from the courtyard below her window, and she lay in bed thinking, "I just want to do something better than him. For a moment."

———

Paul had expanded and refined the health census he'd begun around Cange in 1983. He'd found a book that described a census done in a rural part of India, and he used it as a manual. Ophelia worked on gathering data. This meant walking from village to village, sometimes with Paul, more often with the local youths he had recruited, who knew the ways, down gullies and up mountainsides, along paths half-covered in underbrush. The heat felt "enormous." Her face would turn bright red, but her Creole greatly improved, and every trip seemed important and wrenching. She'd go to a tiny two-room hut, a chair would appear, and the peasants would offer her a drink and talk about their pain and misery while she took notes. She would ask them when they were born, and they would tell her what president had been in power at the time, or date their births to before or after the dam. Ophelia would ask, "How many live here?" and the mother or father of the house would reel off names, sometimes as many as eleven, and Ophelia would look up and see slivers of sky through the banana-bark roof and think about the rainy season. She'd see the metal cups on the stilts of their small granaries and think, "Rats." She noted a distinctive smell inside the crowded huts. "Not smelly socks stinky, but the close smell of people in poverty. Many hungry people breathing."

Sometimes she went to houses where people were dying, and often, especially in Cange among the water refugees, these were children in the throes of one or another of the diarrheal diseases. To get water, the people of Cange had to climb down a steep eight-hundred-foot hillside. They'd dip their calabash gourds or recycled plastic jugs in the stagnant reservoir, then carry them back up the hill, and of course they'd want to make that water last. So it would sit in the jugs or gourds uncovered for days.

The solution came from a team of Haitian and American engineers. The Americans were members of the church group from the Episcopal Diocese of Upper South Carolina who had been helping out Père Lafontant for years. A sparkling underground river burst out near the base of the eight-hundred-foot hill. Before the dam, it had been a main source of local drinking water. The engineers devised a plan to use the force of that river to carry its own water in a pipe up to communal water spigots that would be constructed in Cange. Almost as soon as this was accomplished, Ophelia remembered, infant deaths began dropping.

Farmer was learning about the great importance of water to public health, and he was conceiving a great fondness for technology in general, also scorn for "the Luddite trap." He liked to illustrate the meaning of that phrase with the story of the time when he came back to Cange from Harvard and found that Père Lafontant had overseen the construction of thirty fine-looking concrete latrines, scattered through the village. "But," Farmer asked, "are they appropriate technology?" He'd picked up the term in a class at the Harvard School of Public Health. As a rule, it meant that one should use only the simplest technologies required to do a job.

"Do you know what appropriate technology means? It means good things for rich people and shit for the poor," the priest growled, and refused to speak to Farmer again for a couple of days.

Lafontant was also supervising the construction of a clinic in Cange—the South Carolinians had put up the money. The facility would have a laboratory, of course. Farmer got hold of a pamphlet about how to equip labs in third world places published by the World Health Organization. It made modest recommendations. You could make do with only one sink. If it wasn't easy to arrange for electricity, you could rely on solar power. A homemade solar-powered microscope would serve for most purposes. He threw the booklet away. The first microscope in Cange was a real one, which he stole from Harvard Medical School. "Redistributive justice," he'd later say. "We were just helping them not go to hell."

=

The enterprise in Cange and the surrounding villages was essentially the creation, from scratch, of a public health system, with Père Lafontant as the construction boss—amazing how quickly and durably he got things built in a place without electricity, stores, or a serviceable road. Increasingly, the vision for this health system came from Farmer.

A lot of the plan was straightforward, steps that any school of public health would recommend. He'd begun with the census because that was the way to identify problems and to begin building records and to create a baseline against which future censuses could measure how well the new system was working. He planned for the creation of what he called a "first line of defenses" out in the communities. These would include vaccination programs, protected water supplies and sanitation, and at the heart of the defenses, a cadre of people from the villages trained to administer medicines and give classes on health, to treat minor ailments and recognize the symptoms of grave ones like TB, malaria, typhoid. He imagined his project for women— gynecological services, health education, and family planning—to reduce local maternal mortality. What the first line of defenses failed to prevent would be handled at the second line—at the new Clinique

Bon Sauveur in Cange, which Farmer imagined would someday have a hospital beside it.

To many people in public health, such an array of projects would have seemed ambitious enough, indeed too much to hope for in a place as impoverished as Cange. But by 1985 Farmer had grown impatient with standard definitions of public health. The great burdens of disease in Cange were just a symptom of a general deprivation, he'd say to Ophelia. He'd tell her, "We have to think about health in the broadest possible sense."

This notion came in part from Lafontant. He had built the first school in Cange back in the late 1970s. It had a thatched roof; classes that didn't fit inside were held under a mango tree. In the early 1980s, with money from South Carolina, Lafontant had erected a much larger building, two stories tall, on a small plateau on the hillside above Highway 3. To Farmer the building looked "faintly grandiose," looming above the shacks of Cange. He would write, "The establishment of a school may seem a bit out of place given the homelessness, landlessness, and hunger of many of the water refugees. But it appears that they themselves did not feel that way." Children flocked to the new facility. One peasant woman explained, "A lot of us wondered what would have happened if we had known how to write. If we had known how to write, perhaps we wouldn't be in this situation now." And a school could serve as a place for teaching lessons about health and for providing free meals to malnourished children without injuring their dignity. To build a school was to unite the practical and the moral. Farmer would say, "Clean water and health care and school and food and tin roofs and cement floors, all of these things should constitute a set of basics that people must have as birthrights."

———

All this would require money beyond what the South Carolinians could provide. Farmer had only limited experience as a fund-raiser. In 1985, though, he got lucky.

Two years before, late in 1983, he'd gone to Boston for his standard preadmissions interview at Harvard and had visited a charity named

Project Bread. He'd asked the organization for a few thousand dollars to build a bread oven in Cange. He'd often heard Père Lafontant say that Cange needed a bakery.

It had been an easy sell. Farmer was told that the charity had a donor who had asked that his money go to feed poor people in Haiti.

"Who is he?" Farmer asked.

"He's an anonymous donor."

The bread oven was built, not far from the school, in the summer of 1984. Early the following year, a Harvard Medical School publication printed Farmer's essay "The Anthropologist Within." Soon afterward the director of Project Bread contacted Farmer. The bread oven's anonymous donor had read the article. "I'd like to meet this kid," the donor had supposedly said. "He sounds like a winner."

"If he wants to meet me, tell him to come to Haiti," Farmer replied.

He had been told that the donor's name was Tom White, and that the man owned a heavy-construction firm in Boston. Farmer imagined portly Republicans smoking stogies and cutting back-alley deals with the Massachusetts Bay Transit Authority, keeping the unions out. Farmer went to pick up White at the François Duvalier Airport. The person he found waiting there in the hot wind was a pink-faced man in his sixties, dressed in polyester golfing clothes, including the plaid pants. White had brought along a roll of cash, which he had soon distributed among beggars, not an obnoxious act in Farmer's philosophy but hardly a sufficient one. Farmer narrated Haiti in the truck on the way to Cange, and White seemed appropriately horrified, but Farmer was still wary of him and didn't try to hide the fact.

He was only twenty-five and not, he would admit, "fully formed" when it came to dealing with potential donors. Inside the jouncing truck the conversation turned to American politics. White remarked, "Well, *I* didn't vote for Reagan."

"What do you mean?" said Farmer.

"I didn't vote for Reagan."

"So you voted against your own interests?" asked Farmer.

"Is that a sin?" said White.

Remembering that moment, White told me, "So he went from being cool to very warm." White went on, "He was fresh as hell to me, but I liked him, because if you said boo and he didn't think boo was right, he'd tell you. He was way ahead of me, on service to the poor."

The next time Farmer returned to Cambridge, Tom White took him to lunch, and they had an argument about guilt. White said he thought it was a useless emotion. On the contrary, Farmer said, it could be quite helpful. White had gotten divorced from his first wife. He had made a very generous voluntary settlement with her, and footed all the bills for his children's keep and education. His second marriage—to a woman with six children of her own—was hardly the conventional rich man's. Nonetheless, he said, he felt very guilty about the fact of his divorce.

This wasn't what Farmer had in mind. What he endorsed, he said, was the guilt some rich people felt toward the poor, because it could cause them to part with some of their money. And they *ought* to feel guilty besides.

Actually, White had been giving away money for years, to Catholic charities and needy friends, even before he'd had much of his own. He grew up in an Irish Catholic household devastated by his father's drinking, and at an early age became what he called "the go-to guy" in his family. He'd had a colorful-sounding life. College at Harvard, where he majored in Romance languages, and then the army, where he became, reluctantly at first, the aide to General Maxwell Taylor, commander of the 101st Airborne Division. White parachuted into Normandy the night before D-Day and later into Holland. Though he would say he didn't regret participating, he came away with a hatred for war, and though he liked Taylor personally and admired the general's courage, he learned to dislike the tendency of the powerful to view human beings as pins on a map. Also to dislike the perquisites of power—through seeing a young paratrooper crushed by his own pack, overweight with unnecessary items he carried for the general.

After the war, White had built his father's construction company into what was now the largest in Boston. He had been the intimate of cardinals, had served on the boards of nine institutions, and had sat with the presidential party at JFK's inauguration. But he felt uncomfortable among most of the rich and famous, and generally shunned the press. He told me, cryptically, that he had been depressed at various times in his life. Also that he'd had "a low self-image," adding, "But in my business all you had to be was low bidder." When I asked him what had caused him to place large bets on Farmer, on a medical student in his twenties, White said, "He appealed to me immediately. So intelligent, so dedicated to his work." He thought for a time. "I really can't explain it. I probably was also looking for somebody to hang my hat with."

Certainly Haiti upset White. He found the road to Cange especially offensive. "Jogging along that damn road," he'd say. He never traveled it without thinking, "This would be so damn easy to fix." He remembered his first view of kwashiorkor. "There was a kid with red hair and a bloated belly, and I said right away, 'Put in a feeding program here.'" White found it easy to imagine himself a Haitian. A child with big eyes and a memorable smile, encountered in a dirt-floored hut, made him feel like bringing over the company bulldozers. "For Christ's sake," he'd say to Farmer or Père Lafontant. "Put a tin roof on and pour a concrete floor. I'll give you the money. Holy shit."

When Farmer was back in Boston, doing his internship at the Brigham, White would drive over at lunchtime and buy sandwiches at the restaurant inside the hospital. He and Farmer would eat them in White's car. One day White asked Farmer, who looked pale as usual, "You eatin' enough?"

"Oh, I'm fine," said Farmer.

"Need any money?"

"No," said Farmer. "Well, maybe forty dollars?"

White happened to have a wad of hundred-dollar bills in his pocket. He tossed one into Farmer's lap. "You look hungry to me." Saying this, he felt impelled to reach in his pocket again. He tossed another hundred to Farmer. "Please, for God's sakes, eat," he said, and to emphasize the point, he gave Farmer yet another hundred.

Farmer looked down at the loot. "Now I can tell you what happened last night." He'd gone to the home of an AIDS patient whom he had treated at the Brigham and found out the man was about to be evicted. "I signed my check over to him."

"Jeez, Paul, don't you think that's kind of impractical?"

Farmer smiled. "Well," he said. "God sent *you* today."

White often found himself running errands in Boston for projects in Cange, picking up things like sinks and loading them into the trunk of his Mercedes. (One load of sinks was for a new clinic. The first clinic turned out to have been badly designed. White paid to have it rebuilt. He did this quietly, not asking for credit. "Not even a plaque with his name on it," said Farmer.)

One time when they were together in Boston, White said, "You know, Paul, sometimes I'd like to chuck it all and work as a missionary with you in Haiti."

Farmer thought for a while, then said, "In your particular case, that would be a sin."

CHAPTER 10

In a photograph that Ophelia took in the mid-1980s, Paul appears in shorts, five or ten pounds heavier than in the coming decades—thin but not remarkably so. He crouches, his hands still smoothing the dirt around a seedling he's just planted, on the once barren hillside above Highway 3, where each time she returned Ophelia found another young grove of trees, another new building or two. She came back every summer, from 1985 until 1989. They were months of nearly constant work. By early afternoon Paul would still be seeing patients, and famished herself, she'd go to his office in the clinic. "You're not hungry? All you had was coffee at six this morning." He'd agree to come up the hill to the kitchen with her, but usually reluctantly, she felt.

From time to time she longed to get away from that desolate region. She'd talk Paul into trips to Port-au-Prince, always feeling "sort of scummy" for taking him away. She would tell him, "This is about getting things for the clinic." Before they left she'd grab a handful of his index cards. The drive was a little less than three hours back then. When, as often happened, they punctured a tire or broke a spring and had to wait for repairs, they would sit by the road and she would quiz him. And they would in fact buy medicines and equipment and more flora for Paul to plant around the growing medical complex on the hillside in Cange.

At the end of one of those weekends, they were driving down Delmas Street on their way out of Port-au-Prince, and Ophelia was thinking of the long, hot walks ahead of her in Cange, and of how wonderful it was to return from them and drink a Diet Coke. "I'd love to get some Diet Coke," she said.

Paul said, "We don't have time. We can't do it."

She understood that he wanted to get back to Cange and that making the stop would mean not just a twenty-minute delay but also walking past the beggars into a supermarket that served the Haitian elite. But at the moment, his words nettled her. He seemed to be saying that if he and the peasantry could get along without things like Diet Coke, so could she. "He was so sure about some things," she remembered. "The frustrating thing was, he usually was right." In the car, she started in on him, accusing him of self-righteousness. She didn't let up. Finally, he slammed on the brakes, reached across her, and pushed open her door. "Get out!" he yelled, and called her a foul name. She didn't obey. She sat rigidly in her seat, feeling both offended and also exultant, smiling inwardly, thinking, "*Yes!* I got to you. You have this human quality. You're flawed."

Another trip to Port-au-Prince stood out in her memory. It was in 1986, not long after Baby Doc left Haiti, an event that marked the end of the Duvaliers' reign, which was being followed by what dissident Haitians called Duvalierism without Duvalier, with the Haitian army generally taking on the dictatorial role. All that summer there had been signs of unrest, still rather disorganized: impromptu roadblocks made of burning tires, peasants demonstrating in Mirebalais. A lot of peasants, it seemed, had imagined their lives would improve when Baby Doc left. Now they were protesting the continuation of the status quo. There was, for Ophelia, "a feeling in the air that things could erupt at any moment." She and Paul went to Port-au-Prince for the weekend and were staying at the house that the Lafontants kept in the city. They'd driven downtown on an errand. When they came outside, it seemed to Ophelia that the street had become unusually still, and amid the normal sour odor of the capital she smelled burning tires, "the smell of something being burned that shouldn't be." But kids had taken the keys from their car. While Paul was negotiating with them to get the keys back, Ophelia stared down the street, at its intersection with a larger avenue. Suddenly she saw what in Haiti is known as a *kouri,* literally a run—a stampede of people passing the intersection, and then large Haitian army trucks with mounted guns in close pursuit. She heard shots. The aftermath of a political demonstration, clearly. In a moment demonstrators came running down the street, surrounding their car and all the others that were trying to back and fill and get away from there. She and Paul opened the doors to let in some of the wounded. Meanwhile, she began having stomach cramps. "P.J., let's get out of here!"

Eventually, they got free, and Paul drove to the Lafontants' house. She got out, but he stayed behind the wheel. "I have to go back, Min."

"P.J., please don't."

But he went, right back into the thick of the trouble, demonstrators climbing over the car while soldiers clubbed them. He took several more bloodied civilians in, and came back unbloodied himself. "It was very important to Paul to witness things," Ophelia would say, looking back. She went on, "That smell of burning tires never quite leaves you. The smell is forever associated for me with political violence."

There wasn't much of that out in Cange, but even there the change in atmosphere was obvious. In previous years, before Baby Doc's forced departure, the peasants had rarely dared to talk politics. Now, as a saying went, *baboukèt la tonbe*—the muzzle had fallen off. Farmer would later write, "Not only were the villagers talking about subjects previously forbidden, they were talking about old subjects in new ways." They were no longer merely asking if infant diarrhea was caused by germs but asking whether the germs were caused by dirty water. And didn't dirty water come from the neglect of feckless, greedy governments?

For many years to come, the smell of burning tires, the smell of revolt, of roadblocks and massacres, would be an abiding odor in Haiti, and in Ophelia's life and Paul's.

In 1988 Ophelia came to Boston to live with Paul. By now he had entered the phase of medical school known as clinical rotations, stretches of training at Boston hospitals, usually lasting a month apiece. Paul rarely missed a day of those. But even when he was in Boston, Haiti was never far from his thoughts. He had said to Ophelia when she'd begun working with him in Cange, "We need to bring resources down here. Will you help me?" Back in England after the summer of 1985, she had done some modest fund-raising of her own and, on Paul's instructions, bought ten scales for weighing babies, to use for identifying infants at risk in the continuing health census. She brought the scales and the remaining cash to Cange the following summer.

By then they had begun to talk about creating an organization that would support the growing health system around Cange. Tom White agreed to pitch in, and in 1987 he made the idea real—he hired a lawyer to draw up the papers, creating a public charity in Boston called Partners In Health and a corresponding "sister organization" in Haiti, Zanmi Lasante. Partners In Health would solicit and receive contributions, make them tax-free, and funnel the money, mostly Tom White's, to Cange. White put up a million dollars as what he called "seed money."

Farmer also turned to another well-heeled friend, his old classmate at Duke, Todd McCormack, who was now living in Boston. McCormack was amused at the notion that he, at twenty-eight and working in his father's business, should be on the board of advisers of anything, but he knew Farmer was in earnest and he readily agreed. It seemed to McCormack that, for Paul, PIH wasn't just a stratagem but also a way of trying to create a new communion. "It was a way he could institutionalize what he felt so passionately about, a vehicle through which his friends could participate," McCormack would tell me. "Paul's Catholic church."

Some months after the official founding of PIH, Farmer expanded the group, adding a fellow Harvard anthropology and medical student, a Korean American named Jim Yong Kim. Jim joined PIH after a series of conversations with Paul in Boston, not unlike the long, windy chats Ophelia had with Paul in Port-au-Prince. Farmer offered what for Jim Kim was a convincing vision of the new organization. The reality was less impressive—a charity with a board of advisers and no hired staff except for a bibulous would-be poet, housed in a one-room office above a seafood restaurant in Cambridge. Paul, Ophelia, Jim, and Tom White were most of what there was to PIH, and they spent a great deal of time together. Sometimes the three young people would stay at one of Tom's houses. Tom would go to bed long before they did and in the mornings growl at them, "I don't know what you guys talk about all night long."

They talked about issues such as political correctness, which Jim Kim defined as follows: "It's a very well-crafted tool to distract us. A very self-centered activity. Clean up your own vocabulary so you can show everybody you have the social capital of having been in circles where these things are talked about on a regular basis." (What was an example of political correctness? Some academic types would say to Jim and Paul, "Why do you call your patients poor people? They don't call themselves poor people." Jim would reply: "Okay, how about soon-dead people?")

They talked about the insignificance of "cultural barriers" when it came to the Haitian peasant's acceptance of modern Western medicine: "There's nothing like a cure for a disease to change people's cultural values."

They talked about appearance: "The goofiness of radicals thinking they have to dress in Guatemalan peasant clothes. The poor don't want you to look like them. They want you to dress in a suit and go get them food and water. *Comma.*"

Some people said that medicine addresses only the symptoms of poverty. This, they agreed, was true, and they'd make "common cause" with anyone sincerely trying to change the "political economies" of countries like Haiti. But it didn't follow, as some self-styled radicals said, that good works without revolution only prolonged the status quo, that the only thing projects like Cange really accomplish is the creation of "dependency." The poor were suffering. They were "dying like smelt." Partners In Health believed in sending resources from the

United States to Cange, down "the steep gradient of inequality," so as to provide services to the desperately poor—directly, now. They called this "pragmatic solidarity," a goofy term perhaps, but the great thing about it was that, if you really practiced it, you didn't have to define it, you could simply point at what had been accomplished.

Paul and Jim and Ophelia would go out to dinner, and they'd still be talking about these matters when the restaurants shut down. Then they'd go to Jim's apartment and talk some more. They spent a lot of time defining themselves, rather often by defining what they weren't. WL's were forever saying, "Things aren't that black and white." But some things were plenty black and white, they told each other—"areas of moral clarity," which they called AMC's. These were situations, rare in the world, where what ought to be done seemed perfectly clear. But the doing was always complicated, always difficult. They often talked about those difficulties. How Paul and Jim should balance work for PIH with going to school and getting their degrees. What PIH ought to do next in its adopted piece of Haiti, where AMC's abounded.

≡

Among many other things, they decided to build another school, in a desolate village near Cange—it was called Kay Epin, House of Pines, and it lacked almost everything, including much in the way of trees. Ophelia's father put up the money, three thousand English pounds. On an evening in 1988 Farmer was hurrying around Cambridge, doing last-minute errands before flying to Haiti, where construction of the school was about to begin. He stepped off a curb and got hit by a car. It shattered his knee. So instead of going to Haiti, he went to the Massachusetts General Hospital. He languished there for weeks, then returned in a gigantic cast to the apartment he shared with Ophelia. She tried to nurse him.

Setting up routine housekeeping with Paul hadn't led to a dwindling of affection. "I knew that he loved me. And I loved him," she would say. But for her, relations were strained: "the strain of living with a fellow who was in love with something else, something that I could never compete with, even if I'd wanted to." Often, if he could get away from medical school or his anthropology seminars early on Friday, he'd catch a flight to Haiti for a few days, sometimes just for the weekend. "Please don't go," she said to him on one of those occasions. "Stay with me."

"Come with *me*," he replied.

They argued. He told her, "I was clear about what I wanted to do with my life, and I thought you wanted to join me."

Alone in the apartment afterward, she thought, "It's true. He never said we'd go for walks in the woods, visit art museums, go to the opera."

Everything got more difficult after the accident. Paul was restive in his clumsy cast, and angry because he yearned to get back to his clinic in Cange. She'd remind him he was supposed to keep weight off his broken leg, but he wouldn't listen. She'd cook for him but he wouldn't eat. She did her best, but she didn't suffer silently. They had some rows. Finally, he said to her, "I'm going to Haiti. They don't mind looking after me there."

Years later, she'd still remember the date, December 10, 1988. They would patch up their quarrel, but inwardly she knew something had ended. When he proposed to her a couple of years later, she found it hard to say no but impossible to say yes. Hurt and angry, he told her, "If I can't be your husband, I can't be your friend. It would be too painful."

For a time after that, she got her only news of him through Jim Kim. Away from Paul, her interest in becoming a doctor waned; she really didn't like chemistry. But she hated the separation from Paul. More than ever he seemed to her like an important person to believe in. Not as a figure to watch from a distance, thinking, Oh, look, there *is* good in the world. Not as a comforting example, but the opposite. As proof that it was possible to put up a fight. As a goad to make others realize that if people could be kept from dying unnecessarily, then one had to act. She intended to remain part of PIH, and of Paul's life. She knew he had a great weakness for forgiving people. It was, she thought, the most salient of his priestly qualities. "Gradually I filtered back," she said.

Partners In Health was still being invented, the sort of organization where members could make up their own job descriptions. Once she had filtered back, Ophelia took on PIH's finances and began scheming about creating an endowment. She insisted on being paid a salary, of about fifteen thousand dollars, and yearly contributed three times as much. As for relations with Paul, within a few years they seemed nearly perfect to her. Sometimes when he called her, fresh off the plane from Haiti, after a week or a month away, she'd picture herself his wife, uttering bitter recriminations. But there was none of that now. She simply felt happy at the prospect of seeing him again, and she could tell he felt the same when he appeared in the doorway. "Min!" he'd cry and reach out his arms to her, wearing a wild-looking grin, his face turning bright red. Only his sisters could make him laugh the way she did. It made her feel essential to him when she'd crack a bawdy joke about some mutual acquaintance and see him fall back onto a sofa, scissoring his feet in the air, laughing so hard that his asthma kicked up. He seemed to feel that he could tell her anything, now that he had no formal obligations to her. She'd say to herself sometimes, "Being his wife would have been no bargain. But to be his friend is simply wonderful."

CHAPTER 11

In December 1988, Farmer returned to Cange in a wheelchair, and while his leg mended, he launched his study to improve TB treatment in the central plateau. Big events were happening in Cange, momentous events in Haiti. He witnessed some of those, once his leg had healed, on trips to Port-au-Prince. Several times he was in churches in the capital when shooting started, and he took refuge behind pillars.

Since the departure of Baby Doc Duvalier, various unelected governments had succeeded one another, but it was really the Haitian army that ruled the country from 1986 to 1990—with aid from the United States, as Farmer would discover, searching official, published documents. He was a student of Haitian history, and he knew that trading one corrupt, repressive, and unelected government for another was nothing new for the country or for American policy toward Haiti. Nor were uprisings among the impoverished majority. But it looked to him as though a great popular movement might really be in progress now.

With what seemed like unusual unanimity, the peasants and the people in the slums had embraced something called *dechoukaj,* the "uprooting" of every visible symbol of the Duvaliers, which included the public persecution and sometimes the killing of former *tontons macoutes,* mostly small fry, of course. The reaction of the Haitian army and its paramilitaries was extreme. There was violence on all sides, but as usual the side with guns and money was responsible for most of it. Farmer witnessed some of the incidents and heard about others; later he dug up verification: Haitian army soldiers shooting unarmed demonstrators, entering urban hospitals and threatening staff, sometimes executing patients, even stealing corpses now and then. In 1987 the army's paramilitaries had massacred scores of voters at polling places, aborting what would have been the first democratic elections in Haiti's history.

According to one old saying, perhaps less true by then than formerly, Haiti was 90 percent Catholic and 100 percent Voodoo. (Speaking of a devoutly Christian peasant, Farmer once said to me, "Of course he believes in Voodoo. He just believes it's wrong.") Catholic churches were at the center of the popular revolt—not the cathedrals where the Duvalierist hierarchy presided but what was called *ti legliz,* the small churches of the ruined countryside and of the cities' slums. The most important of these was St. Jean Bosco in Port-au-Prince, where the priest Jean-Bertrand Aristide presided.

Farmer had first heard him speak in 1986, over the radio in Cange. He'd decided to go to Aristide's church and hear him in person. The crowd was rapt, and so was Farmer. Aristide said, as Farmer remembered his words, "People read the Gospel as if it pertained to another place and time, but the struggles described there are in the here and now. The oppression of the poor, the abuse of the vulnerable, and the redemption that comes with fighting for what is right—what ideas could be more relevant in our dear Haiti?" Farmer remembered, "I'd been looking all over for the progressive, liberation theology church in Haiti, and here it was." He joined the crowd that went up to meet Aristide after the Mass. Aristide could hardly have failed to notice him. ("Not many of his parishioners were white, tall, and Creolophone.") They had become friends, but Farmer didn't see much of Aristide in 1988. He was very busy himself in Cange, and Aristide was busy surviving a series of attempted assassinations, including the fire-bombing of his church, which the mayor of Port-au-Prince arranged.

Farmer was hoping for real change in Haiti, and meanwhile hating what he called "the tumble," the turmoil and bloodshed and their inevitable by-product, the worsening of Haiti's already wretched public health. On a day in 1989, he climbed alone to the top of a hill overlooking Cange. In Haiti, he didn't usually write anything except official correspondence and thank-you notes. He didn't usually have time, and besides, writing seemed much less important here than doctoring and building schools and water systems. But he was making an exception on this day, and he climbed the hill to do some work on his Ph.D. thesis in anthropology. "AIDS and Accusation," he'd call it, the first of his alliterative titles.

AIDS had come to Cange about two years after he had, back in 1985. He was writing about its arrival in his thesis. He would catalog what he called "the geography of blame" and the scapegoat role assigned to Haiti. He'd tell the story of how, early in the AIDS epidemic in the United States, sociologists and even medical people had hypothesized that HIV had come from Africa to Haiti, then to the United States. Some experts even hypothesized that the disease had originated in Haiti, where, it was said by some, Voodoo *houngans* ripped the heads off chickens and guzzled their blood, then had sex with little boys. He'd write about how the Centers for Disease Control, a federal U.S. agency, had gone so far as to identify Haitians as a "risk group," along with several other groups whose names began with *h*—homosexuals, hemophiliacs, and heroin users—and about the incalculable harm all this had done to Haiti's fragile economy and to Haitians wherever they lived. In his thesis, he'd marshal a host of epidemiological data to show that AIDS had almost certainly come from North America *to* Haiti, and might well have been carried there by American and Canadian and Haitian American sex tourists, who could buy assignations for pittances in a Port-au-Prince slum called Carrefour.

The thesis was to be an "interpretive anthropology of affliction," combining evidence from ethnography, history, epidemiology, and economics. It would begin, though, with the story of Cange. Following anthropological tradition, he'd give the village a pseudonym, Do Kay. Sitting on the hilltop, on a rocky outcropping, he wrote, "The best view of Do Kay is from atop one of the peculiarly steep and conical hills that nearly encircle the village."

From where he sat, Cange looked like a collection of small dwellings scattered in no particular pattern on the side of an almost treeless mountain. There, near the top, was the house of Dieudonné, empty now because he'd died of AIDS last October. Over there near the road was the house where Anita Joseph had died of AIDS, slowly. A lot of painful memories were incorporated in the landscape. He remembered many other patients who had died, along with their lab data, and remembered vividly three young Haitians who had worked with him on the first health census of Cange: Acéphie, picked off by malaria, Michelet by typhoid, Ti-tap Joseph by puerperal sepsis. Good medicine could have prevented all those deaths. Each friend had died while in the care of doctors, in the typical, substandard Haitian medical facilities that Farmer had come to loathe.

But it wasn't as though failure and death were all he could see from his perch. He could see the clusters of trees that marked the sites of Cange's communal water fountains, connected to the sparkling clean underground river. He could see some of Père Lafontant's communal latrines, which had all but eradicated typhoid in this village. He could see some of the hillside on which Zanmi Lasante had grown and picture the rest—the dormitory and church and the office of the public health project and a corner of the school, and behind the groves of trees he'd planted, the guesthouse, the artisans' workshop, the substantial building that housed the Clinique Bon Sauveur, rebuilt with Tom White's money. And looking back at the village itself, he saw a settlement no longer made of crude lean-tos. Cange had grown, from 107 to 178 households, and the hillside was dotted with little houses now.

Père Lafontant's wife, Mamito, the matriarch of Zanmi Lasante, had supervised a home improvement project, distributing materials that Tom White had paid for and quietly arranging for the reconstruction of the worst of the dwellings. Most of the houses had only two rooms, and many still had dirt floors, but nearly all had roofs of tin, some painted, some rusty, some glinting in the bright sunlight. Six years since he'd first set foot in Cange, and it no longer looked like a miserable encampment of refugees but just a typical, extremely poor Haitian village.

Farmer received his Ph.D. and M.D. simultaneously in the spring of the following year, 1990. His thesis won a prize, and a university press accepted it for publication. Early on certain professors at the medical school—especially the eminent anthropologist Arthur Kleinman and the equally eminent child psychiatrist Leon Eisenberg—had taken a shine to Farmer and licensed his unorthodox habits of attendance. And, as the years went on, they and others would protect him from the enmities and rules of academia. Lives of service depend on lives of support. He'd gotten help from many people.

Farmer's absences from Harvard hadn't hurt his educational standing. For his graduate work in anthropology, Haiti had been a better site than Boston, obviously. And his grades in medical school were outstanding, in part because while studying his flash cards, he'd also worked for large portions of six years as a virtual doctor in Cange. By now, at the age of thirty-one, he'd dealt with more varieties of illness than most American physicians see in a lifetime. He'd also learned how to design and manage both a public health system and a clinic, built from scratch, in one of the most difficult places imaginable, among people whose governments had kept them illiterate, where on a good day concrete got transported by donkey. Not surprisingly, the Brigham and Women's Hospital accepted him into its residency program. It was one of the world's most prestigious, and flexible. A Brigham resident could get permission to pursue another interest. Farmer and Jim Kim, whom the Brigham also accepted, split a clinical residency. Farmer got formal permission, that is, to spend half his time at the Brigham and the other half in Cange.

It seemed possible that Haiti might have a real national election late in 1990. Clearly, though, it wouldn't happen without a fight from the army and the Duvalierist elites and the paramilitaries who worked for them, usually at night. Returning to Cange from Harvard, driving north from Port-au-Prince to Cange, Farmer had to pass through five different military checkpoints. At each, soldiers routinely solicited bribes. Occasionally they confiscated medical equipment that he was bringing to the clinic. Not all the harassment was routine. Zanmi Lasante kept an office in Port-au-Prince. Several times in the months leading up to the election the phone would ring and a voice on the other end would ask for Farmer, then say, for instance, "You are going to be reunited with your granny's bones." He could hear loud clicks on the line when he picked up the phone. Farmer climbed up on the roof of the building, found the bugging device—a clunky-looking jury-rigged thing. Rather gleefully, he kicked it to pieces.

This was all slightly puzzling to him. He hadn't played a visible role in politics. Perhaps he had come to the army's attention because, whenever his patients got arrested, he would go to the jails and try to get them out. Soldiers at the barracks in Mirebalais had shoved him around during two of those attempts at what he called "prison extractions." Or perhaps he cut a larger figure than he realized. It was possible, for instance, that the wrong people had spotted him in the company of Aristide.

In 1990 he saw a lot of the by then famous priest. One day when Farmer happened to be in the city, Aristide stopped by the Zanmi Lasante office, looking bedraggled, driving a white pickup truck with a load of flour for his orphanage in the back. The truck wouldn't start, so he and Farmer loaded the flour into Zanmi Lasante's van and took off. They hit a large puddle, the van stalled, and Farmer said, "I don't think we're going to make it." Then he said to Aristide, "In the newspaper it says you're going to be a candidate for president. I guess they don't know you very well, because you would never run for president."

Aristide said something noncommittal, and a week later declared his candidacy. For a while Farmer felt angry. "How could he participate in something as irremediably filthy as Haitian politics?" But then he thought, "What are the Haitian people saying about this? They're demanding that he run." In a journal Farmer kept during this time, he wrote, "Perhaps this is a singular chance to change Haiti."

Soon he was rooting ardently for Aristide, like virtually everyone else in Cange, and like them listening almost constantly to the radio dispatches from the capital. He was in Port-au-Prince, along with Père Lafontant, on election day. Many foreign observers, including Jimmy Carter, certified the results—67 percent of the vote for Aristide, and only 33 percent for the twelve other candidates. In his journal, Farmer exulted. Haiti had not only the most popular elected head of state in the world but one who professed liberation theology and had promised to lift the country into "dignified poverty." The new president had also promised, not very subtly, a change of fortunes for the Haitian elite. "The rocks in the water don't know how the rocks in the sun feel," said a Haitian proverb. In one of his speeches, Aristide had revised it, saying, "The rocks in the water are going to find out how the rocks in the sun feel."

Farmer drove back to the central plateau the next day. Entering Cange, he spotted an elderly man climbing barefoot up an eroded hillside. Wincing, imagining the man's feet being sliced on the shaley rock—"rocks with teeth," as the local people said—he had a somber thought. "I wondered fleetingly what even a government of saints and scholars could do in the face of such odds," he wrote shortly afterward in his journal. But exultation returned. To Farmer, Aristide wasn't the real victor. It was, he thought, the Haitian peasantry, people like his friends and patients in Cange, who had really won the election. They'd braved intimidation, even massacres, to make it happen and to vote. It seemed as if, at last, after centuries of misery, of slavery and subsequent misrule and foreign interference, the people of Haiti had claimed their country. Nothing, he would later say, had ever moved him so deeply.

He had many reasons to feel hopeful when he went to Boston to put in his time at the Brigham in the summer of 1991. Rumors of coups abounded. One real attempt was aborted. But the new government had assumed power. When he drove to the airport now, he didn't have to stop at army checkpoints and roadblocks. They were gone from National Highway 3. What seemed like a revitalized Haitian Ministry of Health had begun collaborating with Zanmi Lasante on AIDS-prevention work in the central plateau. And at long last it seemed that a real hospital might be built in Cange. Indeed, most of the money had been raised.

On the twenty-ninth of September 1991—a date he wasn't apt to forget—Farmer got Jim Kim to cover for him at the Brigham and set out on a short trip back to Haiti, for a meeting about the new hospital. These days a lot of Boston's cabdrivers, as well as its janitors, were Haitian. The cabbie who picked him up at the Brigham happened to be both Haitian and an acquaintance. As he drove Farmer toward Logan Airport, he said, over his shoulder, "Dr. Polo, there's trouble down there."

"No way," Farmer thought. "This government has the most massive popular support of any in the world." He said to the cabbie, "Don't worry. I'll be in Haiti tonight."

His route was a well-worn path. When he landed in Miami, he went to the usual gate for Port-au-Prince. But the sign above the check-in desk read, CANCELED.

"Whatever for?" Farmer asked the woman at the counter.

"I have no idea," she said.

He checked into a motel near the airport and tuned the TV to CNN, which was just then broadcasting the news that the Haitian army had deposed Aristide. Farmer sat up all night watching, stupefied.

He waited around for flights to resume, then got word that he couldn't take one anyway. The new authorities, the junta, had put his name on a list of personae non gratae. So he returned to Boston. Day after day for two months, he called the Lafontants in Haiti, asking, "Can I come back yet?" Finally, in early 1992, he was told he could. Père Lafontant had bribed a Haitian army colonel to expunge Farmer's name from the list.

When he got off the plane in Port-au-Prince, he was drenched in sweat. He thought, "My pheromones are announcing fear." But he made it through immigration without incident and drove straight to Cange, through the many reconstituted military checkpoints. Two days later he was working in his office at the clinic, beginning to feel calmer, when a former TB patient of his, a young peasant woman with a baby, came in speaking frantically. The local authorities had beaten her husband. He was dying, she wailed. Haitians were always dramatic, though. Imagining a few broken bones, Farmer packed his doctor's bag and went off with her. They hiked across the dam to a hut on the other side of the reservoir.

To protect the victim's family, Farmer would give his patient's husband the pseudonym Chouchou Louis. Later, he'd learn some of the background to the story. While riding in a passenger truck through the central plateau, Chouchou had made a disparaging remark about the state of the road. Inside the truck there was a soldier out of uniform. He overheard Chouchou's *pwen,* his pointed comment, and interpreted it correctly as anti-junta, pro-Aristide. At the next checkpoint, in the town of Domond, soldiers and members of a civilian group called *attachés* hauled Chouchou out of the truck, took him inside the headquarters building, and beat him. Afterward they let him go. But his name went automatically onto a blacklist kept by the local branch of the state's security apparatus. Chouchou lay low for a while, but when he tried to sneak back home, the local section chief and an *attaché* were waiting for him. They had finished their business, and Chouchou was lying on the dirt floor of his hut when Farmer arrived.

He did all he could with the equipment he had in his bag, but even the Brigham's emergency room would probably have failed. Afterward, Farmer recorded the wounds:

> On January 26, Chouchou, a handsome man in his mid-twenties, was scarcely recognizable. His face, and especially his left temple, was misshapen, swollen, and lacerated; his right temple was also scarred, although this was clearly an older wound. Chouchou's mouth was a coagulated pool of dark blood; he coughed up more than a liter of blood in his agonal moments. Lower down, his neck was peculiarly swollen, his throat collared in bruises, the traces of a gun butt. His chest and sides were badly bruised, and he had several fractured ribs. His genitals had been mutilated.

The accounting continued:

> That was his front side; presumably, the brunt of the beatings came from behind. Chouchou's back and thighs were striped

with deep lash marks. His buttocks were hideously macerated, his skin flayed down to the exposed gluteal muscles. Many of these stigmata appeared to be infected.

The people who did this probably weren't far away. Farmer didn't dare go back by the same route, on foot over the dam. He borrowed a canoe, a hollowed-out mango tree, from a local fisherman, and he paddled it back across the lake.

Farmer had to get the story out. He contacted Amnesty International, which added Chouchou's name to a growing list of victims of the junta, and he wrote a piece called "A Death in Haiti," which *The Boston Globe* agreed to publish under someone else's name.

To classmates, later to his students, Farmer's medical memory seemed encyclopedic and daunting, but it was not inexplicable. "I date everything to patients," he told me once. Patients, it seemed, formed not just a calendar of past events but a large mnemonic structure, in which individual faces and small quirks—he'd remember, for instance, that a certain patient had a particular kind of stuffed animal in his hospital room—were like an index to the symptoms, the pathophysiology, the remedies for thousands of ailments. The problem of course was that he remembered some patients all too well. In later years he didn't like to talk about Chouchou. He told me, "I take active precautions not to think about him." By then he'd already described the case in print several times. To me, he simply said, "He died in the dirt."

CHAPTER 12

Ophelia visited Cange during the time of the junta, in the early 1990s. She slept in the main dormitory over the communal kitchen. One morning when she came down to breakfast, Paul said, rather casually, that someone had stood outside his window last night, striking matches.

She'd often felt nervous in Haiti in the turbulent years after Duvalier was thrown out. This was worse. When they ran into soldiers at checkpoints and roadblocks, Paul wasn't even civil to them. He would not take down the iron sculpture that hung in his small room off the clinic, the Aristide symbol of the *kòk kalite,* the fighting "quality" cock. He would leave his books about Che Guevara and Castro and the like unhidden. She thought, "It would be dreadful if they came and searched the place." She lay in bed at night, listening to the dogs barking and the roosters crowing and the drums beating in the hills. One evening she awakened as headlights swept through the louvered windows of her room. The next morning people said that soldiers had been poking around Zanmi Lasante in the night. She thought, "The *plateau central* is the home of the resistance, and there's no way to get out of here, except that road, and everyone knows that this place is full of Aristide supporters." She asked the woman in charge of the kitchen—she was known as Iron Pants, a generic Haitian nickname for a tough woman—"What if they came in to massacre us?"

Iron Pants said, "We'll defend this place with our lives."

Ophelia thought, "With what? Our pots and pans and Culligan watercooler?"

Paul continued to make the edgy transit between Cange and Boston. Indeed, he made it edgier. He asked Tom White to give him ten thousand dollars in cash, which he planned to smuggle into Haiti and turn over to the underground, pacifist resistance. In the car, driving back with the money from Tom's house on Cape Cod, Jim Kim said to Paul, "You're no use to anyone as a martyr." He tried to soften his tone. "If you get yourself killed, Pel, I'm going to kill you."

Paul's face turned bright red. *"What the fuck do you want me to do!"*

Paul had yelled at him before, but Jim had never heard him scream. Paul smuggled the money into Haiti.

Safely back in Boston, Ophelia fretted about him in Cange. He was so angry he might do anything, she thought. What if a soldier came into Zanmi Lasante and tried to arrest one of his patients? "Oh, *God*."

He seemed to be growing more and more reckless. He invited some nuns from the Catholic group Pax Christi to Haiti, hoping they'd help advertise the junta's depredations. Twice at roadblocks, soldiers searched both him and the nuns. One time the soldiers ordered him to get out of the jeep and say, "Long live the Haitian army."

"I'm not going to say that."

"You better say that." They lifted their weapons.

"Okay," he said sweetly.

In Cange, he slept in his clothes, with his shoes on. His room was adjacent to a piece of thickly planted ground, reforested by him. He imagined what he'd do if the soldiers and *attachés* arrived—jump out the window and hide among the vines and trees from the beams of their flashlights. This was morally acceptable, he thought. "Because they'll be coming for me."

Then one day a lone soldier started to enter Zanmi Lasante carrying a gun. Farmer came out to the courtyard. As always, a crowd waited there. "You can't bring a gun in here," Farmer said to the soldier.

"Who the fuck are you to tell me what I can do?"

"I'm the person who's going to take care of you when you get sick," Farmer answered. He was feeling mildly amused, until from the crowd behind him he heard a voice say, *"Ket"*—in rough translation, "Oh, shit." It had the sound of someone anticipating disaster. Farmer thought, "Oh, God, I misjudged the situation." The crowd suddenly seemed like a liability. The soldier couldn't back down in front of them without losing face. But his answer to the soldier was probably the right one, and probably contained the main reason that he wasn't banished or worse during those years. In fact, he was the best doctor in the central plateau, and Zanmi Lasante was the only place where anyone, including soldiers and their families, could get good medical treatment. The soldier growled some menacing words, then left. Farmer's Haitian friends and colleagues scolded him. After that he curtailed his travel. Shots had been fired at Zanmi Lasante's office in Port-au-Prince, and Père Lafontant had decided to close it. Farmer stayed out of the city except when catching planes back to Boston.

He received his MacArthur grant in the summer of 1993, when it seemed that the junta might always be in power. He went to the awards ceremony in Chicago but soon afterward went back to his hotel room—hiding, as he thought of it, and watching the news from Haiti on TV. He was sitting in his room feeling wretched, thinking, "Big deal, I just got a MacArthur. Oh, great. My star's ascending as the Haitians' sets," when he heard voices outside. Haitians! Of course. Who was more likely to be cleaning hotels in the States? He went out and chatted with them, which cheered him up a little.

In Haiti, the body count kept growing. Three close friends of Farmer's had been murdered. He asked Ophelia to give him some money, and he went to Quebec City, his favorite of all cities—he'd always loved snow. In ten days in a hotel room, he wrote 220 pages, most of the draft of a book he would eventually call *The Uses of Haiti*. It is, I think, the best of Farmer's books, certainly the most passionate, essentially a history of American policy toward Haiti. The history, that is, as if written in collaboration with a Haitian peasant.

The perspective is interesting. One learns, for instance, that the United States tried to help the French put down the Haitian revolution in the 1790s and, during the time of American slavery, refused to recognize Haiti and practiced gunboat diplomacy there. Also that, during the American occupation, the U.S. Congress had reconstituted the modern Haitian army and helped to finance it right up until the time when it deposed Aristide; that the head of the junta's death squads, whose minions had murdered Chouchou, had been trained at Fort Benning's School of the Americas; that some of the junta's henchmen and officers in the Haitian army also worked for the CIA; that while formally deploring the coup, Washington, with the help of a generally compliant mainstream American press, was busily denouncing Aristide, even manufacturing lies about him, and maintaining a leaky embargo that seemed calculated to preserve appearances but not to drive the junta out of power.

In the book, a number of heroes don't look so fine. The French revolutionaries, whose idea of *fraternité* didn't include the slaves in St. Domingue, and the Haitian "mulattoes" who went to France to aid those revolutionaries in the hope that they could win the right to own slaves themselves. Woodrow Wilson, who presided over the American invasion of Haiti. Even FDR, who once boasted that, while serving as assistant secretary of the navy, he had written the Haitian Constitution of 1918. (There were others on this list whom Farmer often mentioned elsewhere: the former American slave and great abolitionist Frederick Douglass, who eagerly served as American ambassador to Haiti, in effect representing the Monroe Doctrine there. And Mother Teresa, who came to Haiti in 1981, during the time of Baby Doc, and, as one historian put it, "gushed" over the profligate dictator and his widely hated wife, Michele, who had looted millions from the Haitian treasury for her worldwide shopping sprees. Mother Teresa said Michele had taught her a lesson in humility and marveled at the closeness of the first lady to her people.)

In the United States, there was talk that the new Clinton administration might send troops to put Aristide back in power—albeit with conditions, such as accepting plans for "structural economic adjustment." In early 1994, just before *The Uses of Haiti* came out, Farmer wrote an editorial for *The Miami Herald*. The gist of it was: "Should the

U.S. military intervene in Haiti? We already have. Now we should do so in a new way, to restore democracy." The editorial was mentioned in Haiti, on government radio. Farmer was said to have slandered the Haitian government. Soldiers came looking for him, to escort him out of the country. But he was already in Boston. He was formally expelled again, this time with a finality that even bribery couldn't undo—"I would have expelled me, too, were I them." He moped around the PIH office. Ophelia bought him a guitar, and he actually took some lessons, until the news came that yet another friend had been assassinated in Haiti. Jim half-carried Farmer home, weeping and puking, from a bar that night. The next day Farmer gave away his guitar.

For the rest of the summer of 1994, he lectured about the situation in Haiti to anyone who would listen, in small towns in Maine and Texas, Kansas and Iowa, usually staying at the houses of "church ladies." He testified before a congressional committee along with some nuns—but most of the congressmen were asleep. He debated an American general. "I basically just let it rip," he said later. " 'The Haitian situation is not understandable unless you know that the U.S. created the Haitian army. Blah, blah, blah, infectious disease.' " The general's main response was to yell at him: "Paul, you're totally out in left field!"

Most of the sources Farmer had used in his book were American government documents. He'd imagined that he could merely say he was a doctor and he had written about things he'd either seen with his own eyes or had looked up, and he'd be believed. He was well-received in some quarters, but usually not on the radio. During a show in Fort Lauderdale, a caller said, referring to the boatloads of refugees who were fleeing the poverty and violence in Haiti and trying to get to Florida, "We can't have Haitians coming into our country."

"Why not?" Farmer said. "*My* family are boat people."

The host, understandably, didn't get it. "Dr. Farmer, are you Haitian?"

Several times, and especially after the general yelled at him, he thought, "Screw this. I want to go back to my clinic." He returned the day after Aristide was reinstated as president, in mid-October 1994.

=

The three years of military rule in Haiti had resembled a war, and like every war produced a public health disaster. The United Nations estimated that about eight thousand people got killed, most of them murdered by the Haitian army and its paramilitaries. Many boat people, perhaps thousands, drowned while trying to get away, and more died than on the *Titanic* when a leaky old ferry named the *Neptune* had sunk. But deaths from drowning and gunshots and torture probably made up just a fraction of the total. There was no telling precisely how much public health had deteriorated by the time military rule ended, but Farmer could make some guesses, based on the wreckage he returned to in Cange.

Somehow Père Lafontant had managed to get the new hospital built. But all Zanmi Lasante's projects in the villages around Cange had been interrupted—its programs for women's literacy, for vaccinating children, for sanitation and clean water, for distributing condoms and other AIDS-prevention measures. Partners In Health had financed a movie about HIV. Patients created the script, which depicted a truck driver and a soldier romancing several female victims. It was being shown to a crowd in a village school when soldiers walked in and shut down the projector. Not the wisest thing, during the reign of a military junta, to show a movie that blames AIDS on soldiers. Zanmi Lasante had put the movie away for the duration.

In the region, only Zanmi Lasante had dared to treat people who had been beaten or shot. The army had shut down the clinic once, briefly. The place was marked. Afraid to be seen there, afraid to travel at all, lest they end up like Chouchou, many patients hadn't come until they'd grown very ill. Many had simply stayed away. The number of patients fell by half during those years, yet the clinic recorded an annual doubling of injuries from assaults—including four rapes committed by soldiers and *attachés*—a large increase in typhoid, and twenty-two times more cases of measles than the average before the coup. The years of military rule had exacerbated the chronic malnutrition, and tuberculosis had risen markedly in the region. The junta had focused most of its terror on the urban slums, because some of Aristide's most ardent support was concentrated in them, and the slums were also at the center of Haiti's AIDS epidemic. Hundreds of thousands fled back to the countryside. At Zanmi Lasante, in 1993, the number of patients with AIDS had increased by about 60 percent.

Several of the staff had resigned in fear. Farmer wrote that "paralysis" and "lassitude" afflicted almost all the medical personnel who stayed on. They missed meetings or canceled them, abandoned research, found excuses for not resuming the interrupted projects. Haitian doctors, he'd long ago discovered, learned early to accept all sorts of deficiencies—shortages of medicines, filthy hospitals. Perhaps it is a universal tendency to view the deaths of strangers philosophically. Haitian doctors had better cause for this failing than most others in medicine. Not surprisingly, they tended to shrug when patients died from ailments like measles or tetanus or TB. Farmer had put some of his best efforts into teaching his staff to expect more of themselves. Now many were shrugging again.

But the situation was far from hopeless, and he was glad to be back.

═══

Farmer was thirty-five now, on the rise in both medicine and anthropology. He had won his MacArthur. He was an infectious disease fellow in training at one of the world's best teaching hospitals, an assistant professor in medical anthropology at Harvard, and the author of two books and about two dozen articles. He seems to have looked forward to a great deal more of the same, and he seems to have imagined that his main jobs now, and PIH's as well, were to repair Zanmi Lasante and keep expanding it.

Partners In Health had changed their offices twice since 1987. They had finally acquired their own small headquarters building in Cambridge—the idea had been Jim Kim's, the money Tom White's. The staff there numbered only about a dozen, a little less than half volunteers, the rest underpaid employees. They managed an AIDS-prevention program for Haitian teenagers in Boston and, in the run-down neighborhoods right next to the Brigham, a program for providing medical and social services to people who weren't getting any. They supported, with small sums and advice, a few public health projects in far-flung places, such as Chiapas in Mexico, and their research branch, dedicated to criticizing the status quo in international health, was assembling a book about the special worldwide vulnerability of impoverished women to AIDS. (*Women, Poverty, and AIDS,* it was called. Hearing the title, a friend of Farmer's said, "That's what I like about your books, Paul. They have such cheerful subjects.") One could hardly have called PIH Paul's Catholic church anymore, but for all their cosmopolitan outlook, they were still just a small public charity with a substantial medical complex in Haiti, and Farmer seems to have felt they were going to stay that way. In PIH's 1993 annual report, he'd written that they should never change their mission or soften their message in order to broaden their appeal. Accordingly, he wrote, they should resign themselves "to a somewhat marginal status."

But, in fact, a big change in PIH was about to begin. They were about to become players in international health.

Part III

—

Médicos Aventureros

A simple epidemiological map, a map based on what makes people sick and what kills them, and in what numbers and at what ages, could be coded in two colors. One would stand for populations who tend to die in their seventies, mainly from illnesses that seem like inevitable accompaniments to the aging of bodies. The other color would stand for groups who, on the average, die ten and even forty years earlier, often from violence and hunger and infectious diseases that medical science knows how to prevent and to treat, if not always to cure. On this map, the line dividing the two color-coded parts of humanity—what Farmer called the "great epi divide" (*epi* being short for *epidemiological*)—would partition many countries, many cities. Most of Haiti would wear the color of ill health, but parts of the hills above Port-au-Prince would be a patch of well-being. The map of the United States, by contrast, would depict a healthy nation speckled with disease. In Boston's Mission Hill neighborhood, right next to the Brigham, for instance, infant mortality is higher than in Cuba. In New York City's Harlem, a famous study from 1990 showed, death rates for males between the ages of five and sixty-five were higher than in Bangladesh.

Meager incomes don't guarantee abysmal health statistics, but the two usually go together. Many of the groups of people living on the wrong side of the great epi divide have brown or black skin. Many are female. What they all have in common is poverty. Absolute poverty, the lack of almost every necessity—clean water and shoes, medicine and food—in a place like Haiti. Relative poverty in a place like New York.

For Farmer and Jim Kim and many others interested in the distribution of disease, tuberculosis vividly illustrated the great epi divide, its contours, its causes, its effects. Improperly treated, or not treated at all, TB is dreadful and lethal, usually devouring the lungs but also sometimes other organs, and sometimes the bones. Fortunately, an array of good and inexpensive "first-line" TB drugs existed. They had to be administered over the course of months—usually six to eight months—but then they cured virtually every case. Thanks in part to those antibiotics, tuberculosis had all but vanished from the rich parts of the world. But the disease still plagued the poor parts to a degree most Americans and many western Europeans would find hard to credit. At the end of the twentieth century, TB was still killing about two million people a year, more adults than any other infectious disease, except for AIDS, and TB shared what Farmer called "a noxious synergy" with AIDS, since an active case of one often makes a latent case of the other active, too. In poor countries, TB was the most common proximate cause of death among people who died with AIDS. And yet, because tuberculosis mainly afflicted the poor side of the epi divide, the industrial nations and pharmaceutical companies had all but abandoned the search for new technologies to fight it. The tools for diagnosing the disease were antique; no large campaign had been launched to find a fully effective vaccine; and the newest of the antituberculous drugs had been developed twenty-five years ago.

Farmer liked to say that tuberculosis made its own preferential option for the poor. The aphorism contained a certain literal truth. According to the best current estimates, about two billion people, one-third of humanity, have TB bacilli in their bodies, but the disease tends to remain latent. It multiplies into bone-eating, lung-consuming illness in only about 10 percent of the infected. The likelihood of getting sick increases greatly, though, for those who suffer from malnutrition or various diseases, especially from HIV, itself by now predominantly a disease associated with poverty. Usually, active TB feeds on the lungs and spreads itself from them, sneezes and coughs like the wind to its seeds. People who live in crowded peasant huts and urban slums and shantytowns and prisons and homeless shelters stand the best chances of inhaling the bacilli, of having their infections expand into active disease, and in some settings, of getting just enough treatment to make their TB drug-resistant.

A person with active TB of the lungs harbors hundreds of millions of bacteria, enough to ensure that a small number will be mutants impervious to anti-TB drugs. In a patient who gets only one antibiotic or inadequate doses of several, or who takes the medicines erratically or for too short a time, the drug-susceptible bacilli may die off while the drug-resistant mutants flourish. The patient becomes a site of rapid bacterial evolution, with drugs supplying the selective pressure. In the gravest cases, patients end up infected with bacilli that can't be killed by the two most powerful drugs. Medical science reserves a special name for tuberculosis of that sort—multidrug-resistant TB, MDR by abbreviation. It is a scary disease, and a serious problem wherever it appears, but worst, of course, in the places with the fewest resources to deal with it.

=

Multidrug-resistant TB tends to arise where wealth and poverty are mingled, where poor people get some treatment but not enough. It arises only infrequently in places of nearly universal poverty like Haiti, where most people don't get treated at all. But by the mid-1990s Farmer had dealt with several cases of MDR in Cange. The first had appeared during the time of the junta. He remembered the feeling of dread that washed over him when he realized what his patient had. And dread was justified; the young man died.

Farmer blamed himself, but the fact was that treating MDR was tricky under the best of circumstances, and for a while, during the time of the junta, he simply couldn't get the necessary medicines to

Cange. Since the death of that patient, he'd assembled the resources to fight the disease at Zanmi Lasante, both the tools and the procedures. He was curing most of the cases that appeared sporadically in Cange when, in 1995, MDR claimed a close friend who had been living in a shantytown on the outskirts of Lima, Peru.

CHAPTER 14

For several years during medical school, Farmer had boarded at St. Mary of the Angels, a parish run by a priest known as Father Jack. Farmer camped in a room under the eaves of the rectory. The church was in Roxbury, one of Boston's run-down neighborhoods, largely African American. In the musty, dim, low-ceilinged sanctuary, gospel music surrounded the Mass, and sermons had the feel of revival meetings. Jack Roussin, the priest, a beefy man with a florid complexion, would declaim on poverty and injustice, voices in the congregation calling out amens.

Jack was the kind of priest whom nervous bishops call "a character." He mediated arguments among neighborhood gangs, led candle-light vigils against drug dealing, carried signs in front of the State House protesting cuts in welfare. In his spare time, he liked to tell off-color stories and tease the young medical student upstairs. When Farmer began practicing vivisection—dog lab it was called at the medical school—he had a long talk with Jack about his misgivings, working on a creature he was going to have to kill. The next morning Farmer awoke to what sounded like fingernails scratching on his door, then imitations of whinings, finally a few howls. Ophelia stayed at the rectory sometimes. She'd muss up the sheets in the room the nuns assigned her, then cross herself as she crept up the stairs to Paul's garret. Father Jack pretended not to notice, but he'd talk about Farmer's previous girlfriends in front of Ophelia just to see Paul blush. When

Farmer created Partners In Health, he put Father Jack on the board of advisers.

In the early 1990s, Jack left St. Mary's for a church in a place called Carabayllo, a slum on the outskirts of Lima, Peru. On visits back to Boston, he kept telling Paul and Jim and Ophelia that PIH should start a project down there in his new parish.

Jim Kim agreed, eagerly. For about eight years Jim had happily served—very happily, he insisted—as Paul's second in command or, as one member of the organization put it, PIH's *bayakou,* Creole for a person who picks up excrement. He'd answered the phone at PIH, helped Paul get medicines and appliances for Zanmi Lasante, written grant proposals. When Paul had to get from the Brigham to a meeting, it was Jim who made sure he got there on time and who would escort him out of the hospital, saying, "Okay, Pel, we're in a hurry. Only one hug and two kisses per janitor." Now Jim wanted to do more. He wanted to learn how to do what Paul had done in Haiti.

Farmer wasn't enthusiastic, but once he gave in, he did everything he could to help. First of all, he talked Tom White into putting up thirty thousand dollars, half the initial cost of the project. And Farmer gave Jim advice and encouragement almost daily, often in phone calls between Lima and Cange.

Jim planned to imitate a part of Zanmi Lasante. He'd create a system of community health workers in Carabayllo which they'd call Socios en Salud—a Spanish version of Partners In Health. He imagined a small health improvement project, but he wasn't thinking small. He wasn't capable of that. He envisioned a project so well-designed and managed that it would inspire imitation in other periurban slums all over the world. In photos from around this time, Jim appears as a neatly groomed, well-proportioned young man, a few inches shorter than Farmer, with jet black hair swept into a knifelike wave, and wire-rimmed glasses over narrow eyes. He had an expressive face. His eyes would disappear completely when he grinned. He talked fast, and he radiated intensity, especially at this moment. He was excited. He wrote a letter to Father Jack. "I have purchased the three-volume Pimsleur tape system and have committed myself to learning as much

Spanish as I can as quickly as I can. Are there any books that you would recommend on Peru?" Almost as soon as he got to Lima, Jim started placing long-distance calls to Paul.

"Pel, you won't believe what Father Jack just did. He's hiring all these people because he feels sorry for them, and they *can't do the work.*"

Paul would answer calmly. "Don't confront Jack. You're new there. Just keep on working."

Various leaders in Carabayllo asked Socios to build a pharmacy, which would dispense free medicine to the most impoverished people in the slum. Socios erected the pharmacy right next to Father Jack's church. But Peru was in the midst of a civil war, between the government and the Shining Path guerrilla movement. Some of the guerrillas, it was said, used Carabayllo as a bedroom, and they had their own ideas about what was best for the slum. On midnight on New Year's Eve, while Jack was saying Mass, the pharmacy blew up. The church had a bank of glass front doors, but Jack liked to preach with them open, so none of the glass flew inward at the congregation. Word got back that guerrillas had planted the bomb because the pharmacy represented "crumbs for the poor," a palliative designed to curb the growth of revolutionary fervor. Paul and Jim received the news philosophically. As a matter of fact, they *were* dispensing palliatives, they said. Partners In Health simply had the pharmacy rebuilt, in a different spot. There were many frustrations, small and large, many occasions when Jim felt insulted. Paul would tell him: "Remember, serving the poor in Carabayllo is more important than soothing your own ego. It's called eating shit for the poor." This sort of advice was always tonic for Jim. He'd feel as though catastrophe loomed, he'd call Paul and tell him about the problem, and Paul would say sympathetically, "Yeah, I remember something like that happened three times in Cange."

Farmer also traveled to Lima, to conduct a health census in the slum, as Ophelia had helped him to do a decade ago in Cange. He found many of the same kinds of problems there, but none as acute. Naturally enough, after all his years in Haiti, he wondered if tuberculosis was a problem in Carabayllo. It had been, he learned. For a long time TB control in Peru had been haphazard, but the country had recently created a nationwide program. They'd done this with advice and assistance from the World Health Organization—WHO, a branch of the United Nations. Its pronouncements carry a lot of weight in poor countries, and WHO had declared Peru's new TB control progam the best in the "developing" world. The praise seemed justified to Farmer when he read the official data. He'd remember, a bit ruefully, telling Jim, "The one thing we don't need to do here is TB."

Then Father Jack got sick. In May 1995 he flew to Boston, and Jim drove him to the Brigham, where the doctors diagnosed tuberculosis. The Brigham doctors put Jack on a standard regimen of four first-line TB drugs, a virtually foolproof cure in most locales. But Jack died about a month after starting therapy. A sample of his TB survived him, in a culture at the Massachusetts State Lab, where it was being tested for drug susceptibility. The results arrived a day or two after Jack's death. They showed that the bacilli from his body were resistant to all four of the drugs he'd been given, and to the one other first-line drug as well.

=

On the plane to Lima for the memorial service, Farmer wondered aloud to Ophelia, over and over, what he should have done to save Jack. In the hotel room after the ceremony, it seemed as if Paul would never stop weeping. When they went down to dinner and the waiter asked if they wanted to sit in the no-smoking *zona,* Jim said, "How about a no-cry zone?" And Paul kept on crying but started laughing as well.

Sentiment and remorse became a goad. But the clinical facts of Jack's death were the real issue. They altered Farmer's view of Jim's project. Before, he'd felt that if Jim really needed to do his own thing, Carabayllo made for a reasonable site, another needy place where PIH could help. Now it seemed likely that they'd happened on something much more complicated, also more significant, and maybe even frightening. Father Jack had never before been treated for TB, so there was only one way he could have contracted a five-drug-resistant strain. He had to have caught it from someone else, most likely in Carabayllo.

Back before Father Jack's death, while helping Jim on the health census, Farmer had asked the project director of Socios en Salud if drug-resistant tuberculosis was a problem in the northern slums of Lima. The director—his name was Jaime Bayona—had examined the official records and found nothing. He'd decided to look further, though. He'd gone to various public clinics and asked the doctors and nurses if they had any patients with highly resistant strains. Invariably they said they did not. But often, Jaime noticed, they paused before answering. So he started asking his question in a different way: "Did you have any TB patients who came and were treated but weren't cured?"

"Oh, sure," one nurse had replied, and had proceeded to introduce him to an impoverished woman from Carabayllo named Señora Brigida. Jaime visited her. She told him her story. A government clinic had treated her for TB, but she had relapsed. Her second course of therapy had been interrupted by a strike of medical workers—the government of Alberto Fujimori had cut social service spending drastically, and the health workers had gone out in protest. Eventually her TB had been cultured and found to be resistant to four first-line drugs. She'd been re-treated again—with those very same drugs, strangely enough—and now she was sick again and coughing blood. Along the way doctors had accused her of "noncompliance," and her son had died of TB, more than likely from a strain of the disease that he'd caught from her. Jaime had related the story to Farmer in the Lima airport just before Paul caught a flight to Miami. Farmer had promised to find the drugs to treat Señora Brigida, and he'd pondered her case, looking down at Lima from the airplane. If drug-resistant TB was abroad in the crowded shantytowns, he reasoned, it would spread across that sprawling city. He thought, "The Peruvian authorities are going to have to pay attention to this."

But it seemed to Jaime Bayona that they were doing something like the opposite. Jaime was Peruvian. He'd been an altar boy for a priest friend of Father Jack's and had earned a degree in public health. Jim had recruited him to direct Socios. Jim had liked him at once—this small, quiet man in his thirties, a man of understated smiles, always neatly dressed, always pushing his glasses back up onto the bridge of his nose. In the aftermath of Jack's death, Jaime stepped up his visits to the government clinics. He'd ask his question, and sometimes a nurse would bring out a stack of medical records and open them, saying, "We have something here that might interest you, but I can't show it to you."

And Jaime would say, "Okay, fine." He'd push his glasses back into place and stare across the desk at the opened files. Soon he'd taught himself to read patients' records upside down. Again and again he read stories of patients who hadn't been cured by standard chemotherapy, or by repeated retreatment with first-line drugs. He'd saunter out of the health centers, then drive as fast as he could to the Socios office in Carabayllo, a concrete building that belonged to Father Jack's church, now named the Father Jack Roussin Center. He'd hurry inside, sit down at his computer, and type up what he'd read, in e-mails addressed exclusively to Farmer and Kim.

CHAPTER 15

I first saw Carabayllo at night, in Farmer's company. The road from the airport, four lanes and divided, felt very smooth, even after the driver turned away from the old Spanish colonial center and the skyscrapers of downtown and headed into the settlements of Lima's northern outskirts. In the median, palm trees rustled past. I gazed out the car window at hillsides smothered in darkness but dotted with twinkling lights, as if by Japanese lanterns, pretty in the night. "Lima doesn't seem like the third world," I said.

"Oh, yes it is," said Farmer. "You'll see."

Lima is a vast coastal city, vast and dry. In the daylight the northern neighborhoods seemed like an endlessly spreading slum, the roads choked with traffic and with motorcycle rickshaws and minibuses that served as public transportation, and the banks of the roads littered with broken-down vehicles and garbage, and garbage on fire, and with ramshackle-looking development, like American strip malls that had moldered before being completed. On cement-block walls, there were signs for bars and nightclubs and hairdressers and, everywhere it seemed, for doctors, with the prices for office visits painted on the walls. In the gloomy air of daytime Lima—the sun filtering down through thin fog from the Pacific, then through the perpetual ground-level strata of dust and hydrocarbons—I stood outside Socios headquarters and looked up toward Carabayllo's hills and realized that the lights I'd seen the night before were mounted on highway-style pylons, towering over one- and two-room shacks. The hovels were perched on the sides of steep, gray-brown hills—giant heaps of sand and rock and nothing growing on them, except for the shacks and a few little gardens beside them and those weirdly outsize light poles.

Many of the people in Carabayllo came from Andean villages. They had jet black hair and high cheekbones. When he first saw them trudging up and down these hills, which they themselves compared to the surface of the moon, even Farmer, with all his firsthand knowledge of Latin American poverty, felt viscerally puzzled. He thought of the places the settlers had left behind, imagining pictures of wild green mountains in coffee table books about the Incas. Looking up at the electric pylons, though, he guessed their reasons. People he talked to told a familiar story, like stories he'd heard from peasants who had migrated to the slums of Port-au-Prince. They had come to Carabayllo in the hope of finding things their hometowns didn't have: electricity, clean water, schools, medical care, and jobs, also distance from the war between the Shining Path and the Peruvian army.

On one side of Carabayllo, on the lowland beside the road, there were stores, garages, vendors' carts, kiosks roofed with umbrellas, and, on side streets and the lower hillsides, thick clusters of small houses made of brick and concrete. The light poles and paved roads ascended the hills. The pavement turned to dirt, then roads turned into paths, and the houses grew more and more provisional. Scattered among them, there were dirt-floored convenience stores, metal-roofed cook shacks (where residents bought dinner because they couldn't afford stoves and the fuel for stoves), barbershops, even graveyards. The air carried a strengthening smell of urine. There were no sewers up there, the only bathrooms secluded places among the boulders above the last dwellings. I looked out to the north. In the distance I could see a river, a line of green, but all around and high above only dirt and rocks. A couple of children were playing nearby with a ball. It got away from them. I watched the ball bounce downhill until I lost sight of it, thinking of gravity, sewage, and disease.

On these hillsides and down in the lowlands, Jaime Bayona had found, rather quickly, ten Carabayllanos with probable MDR. To confirm the diagnosis, samples of each patient's TB had to be regrown in cultures and tested for drug susceptibility. The general procedure was more than a century old, but beyond the reach of many of the places in the world with the greatest burdens of TB. Peru's national lab could do the work, but Socios didn't have access to it. Farmer solved the problem as he'd long since solved it in Haiti, where he couldn't get cultures done either. He took specimens from those ten patients and packed the jars in his suitcase, eventually depositing them at the Massachusetts State Lab outside Boston. He labeled the jars "Paul Farmer, TB Commissioner"—he was in fact a member of a state TB commission. He enjoyed these transnational diagnostic excursions, for him small acts of redistribution. But the results of the cultures were alarming. When it comes to treating MDR, every drug lost to resistance makes a cure more difficult and expensive, and most of the ten patients in Carabayllo had TB resistant not only to the two most powerful drugs but to all five of the first-line antibiotics, just like Father Jack. In Farmer's experience, such severe resistance patterns were unusual, but here it seemed as if they might be the norm, and he wondered why.

Farmer flew from Haiti to Lima, and Jaime Bayona took him straight from the airport to a small health clinic, run by the government, at the base of the Carabayllo hills next to Father Jack's former church, Cristo Luz del Mundo. A sign on the wall outside the clinic read EL PROGRESO. It was a dusty little concrete building with a small cabinet of medicines in a corner—most bathrooms in American homes were better stocked. The ten patients were awaiting the American doctor inside.

Farmer sat on a wooden bench, his stethoscope around his neck, and Jaime sat beside him, to act as interpreter—Farmer couldn't yet speak Spanish. One after the other, the ten patients came in and sat down on a bench in front of Farmer. Some were so sick they had to be carried in. He studied their chest X rays—the outlines of the encysted cavities, swarming with bacilli, that TB had formed in the lungs of many; the extensive infiltrates that appeared as streaks of white, like cirrus clouds, against a black background; the voids where TB bacilli had eaten the upper lobes of lungs. He listened to their chests through his stethoscope, plugging his ear into their lungs as it were, hearing the crackles known as rales—the sounds of alveoli pulling open against fluid—and the prolonged wheezings called rhonchi—the patient's breath rushing through narrowed airways.

Farmer was a TB expert. When he was still just a resident at the Brigham, he'd written a treatment manual for the house staff. He had been diagnosing and treating the disease ever since he'd first set foot in Haiti, where nearly everyone was infected and active cases were rampant. Now, as he studied the ten patients' records, he was aware of a difference from the Haitian norm. In Cange his MDR patients usually told stories of therapy interrupted, by a strike or a flood or the abrupt closing of a clinic. Stories, that is, of severe resistance arising from too little medicine. These ten patients from Carabayllo had a different kind of case history. They'd received free treatment daily, under the auspices of the national TB program, strictly in accordance with the guidelines published by WHO. They'd undergone what the World Health Organization called DOTS. The initials stand for directly observed treatment short-course chemotherapy, a very effective and inexpensive strategy, the same strategy Zanmi Lasante had been using for years. Farmer called DOTS the most significant advance in TB control since the advent of antibiotics. He applauded WHO's plan to spread it all over the world. But here in Carabayllo, for these ten patients at least, something had gone wrong.

The first round of DOTS hadn't cured them. When that happened, WHO guidelines called for retreatment with the same antibiotics, plus one. This prescription came from clinical trials in Africa, where it had worked well. In those trials it had seemed that most treatment failures arose because of patients' noncompliance—because they hadn't taken all their pills, not because they were infected with highly drug-resistant strains. So when a patient failed standard therapy, it seemed reasonable to try again, by merely strengthening the regimen a little and making sure all the doses were taken.

But the African studies were more than twenty years old, and Peru wasn't Africa. For one thing, Peru hadn't used the same drugs during its period of chaotic TB control. And dusty little clinic though this was, it had done its job properly. Farmer felt sure of that. The patients' records showed they'd swallowed their pills under the direct observation of nurses and aides. Through Jaime, Farmer asked them, one after the other, if they'd taken all their doses. When they answered, saying that they had, he stared at their eyes. He'd been a doctor long enough, he felt, to sense a lie. He believed these people. Three were themselves health workers. They knew what pills they were supposed to take, and they, too, claimed they'd followed doctors' orders.

Farmer leafed through their records, Jaime leaning over his shoulder, translating. These ten people had all been sick a long time. They'd been treated with DOTS, then treated again, and many had undergone further retreatments, and now all of them had four- and five-drug resistance. In his mind, Farmer reviewed the possible explanations. He'd already ruled out noncompliance, he felt, and poor drug quality couldn't be blamed—international experts had certified the drugs' efficacy. And these patients couldn't have caught the same highly resistant strain, because each one's TB had a slightly different pattern of resistance.

There was one other possibility. Suddenly, suspicions that had been forming in Farmer's mind seemed likely, indeed inescapable.

The dynamics of tuberculosis make it nearly impossible for a person to acquire resistance to more than one drug at a time, but repeated improper therapy can select for increasingly resistant mutants and create strains resistant to any number of drugs. This was what must have happened to these ten people, Farmer thought. They had gone to the clinics with one- or, more likely, two-drug resistance, and through treatment and repeated retreatment under the standardized DOTS formulas, they had emerged with four- and five-drug resistance. The biological principles were elementary. It wasn't as if Farmer imagined that he had come up with new science. But for a moment, sitting on the bench in the clinic, the pieces falling together in his mind, he felt an old familiar pleasure. The motion of his mind toward root causes had always excited him. He loved the challenge of diagnosis and all its accoutrements—the stains on the microscopic slides, the beautiful morphologies of the creatures under the lens. But what he called "the eureka moment" had a bad aftertaste this time. Later he would tell me, "God, I'd hate to ever feel triumphant about something so rotten."

There was a proper procedure for dealing with resistance. When a patient didn't get better on standard therapy, a doctor should suspect that the TB was impervious to some drugs in the regimen and should find out which drugs as quickly as possible and substitute others. Giving patients the wrong drugs was both useless and dangerous. It could lead to what infectious disease specialists call "recruitment of further resistance." The term exactly described the process that Farmer saw in the ten patients' records. He chose to call the process "amplification," because that term sounded worse. These ten Peruvians had gone to the doctor sick and emerged, about two years later, sicker, their TB becoming resistant to more and more drugs as it went on eating their lungs. Not because they hadn't followed doctors' orders, but precisely because they had. And those orders weren't simple acts of stupidity or carelessness. They were enshrined as official policy. They came from on high, from the people in charge of Peru's TB program, who had gotten them from Geneva, from the World Health Organization itself.

The story, as Farmer pieced it together, became increasingly painful. After amplifying resistance in these ten patients, the national program had essentially abandoned them. Tuberculosis patients could consult private pulmonologists, but they had to pay for the visits and for the very expensive second-line drugs the pulmonologists prescribed. Farmer and Kim and Bayona would soon meet people whose families had sold most of their meager possessions and had bought as much of those drugs as they could. Not enough to get cured, however, only enough to acquire still further resistance. Others had given up and gone back to their shacks on the barren, dusty hillsides and were waiting there to die.

In effect, WHO had prescribed this for them, too. The official DOTS manual contained the following statement: "In settings of resource constraint, it is necessary for rational resource allocation to prioritise TB treatment categories according to the cost-effectiveness of treatment of each category." Farmer and Kim began collecting a number of official WHO statements. Some put the case more plainly: "In developing countries, people with multidrug-resistant tuberculosis usually die, because effective treatment is often impossible in poor countries."

For Farmer, and for Jim and Jaime, there was a larger principle involved. A TB epidemic, laced with MDR, had visited New York City in the late 1980s; it had been centered in prisons, homeless shelters, and public hospitals. When all the costs were totaled, various American agencies had spent about a billion dollars stanching the outbreak. Meanwhile, here in Peru, where the government made debt payments of more than a billion dollars every year to American banks and international lending institutions, experts in international TB control had deemed MDR too expensive to treat.

CHAPTER 16

Peru had established its rigorous TB program, its model WHO program, only four years back, in 1991. This was after decades of inadequately financed and unsupervised treatment, which had spawned drug-resistant strains. It seemed likely to Farmer that these had spread fairly widely. Jaime Bayona had already turned up dozens of probable cases, and he had done this working alone, reading records upside down. So while they didn't know exactly how many people in the slum had MDR, Kim and Farmer felt pretty sure that there would be more than a handful, more than the ten Jaime had brought to the clinic for Farmer to examine. And the prospect of treating more than a handful was daunting.

Some time ago, when he'd first encountered MDR in Haiti, Farmer had gone to a man named Michael Iseman for advice. Iseman was the world's foremost clinical authority on the disease, and he worked in the world's best MDR treatment center, National Jewish in Denver. And yet in 1993 he and his colleagues had reported cure rates of only about 60 percent and costs that had run as high, in one especially difficult case, as $250,000. The disease was hard to treat anywhere, and bound to be harder, if less costly, in Carabayllo than Denver. The main tools, the so-called second-line drugs, would have to be imported. They were very expensive. Some were scarce. All were weak and had nasty side effects, which a patient had to endure for about two years—in the best case, stomachaches and months of intramuscular injections; in the worst, hypothyroidism, psychosis, and, if the doctor wasn't careful, even death. Most of the patients in Carabayllo would be impoverished. Most would need not just drugs and careful monitoring but encouragement and food and new roofs and water pipes.

Paul and Jim and Ophelia talked again and again, in Boston and on airplanes and by e-mail, about whether they should take on this problem. But there really wasn't much question of turning away. Jim took an expansive view: "Forgive me for saying this, but the great thing about TB is that it's airborne." Tuberculosis was only predominantly a disease of the poor, Jim reasoned. Others got it, too, just from breathing. In the era of AIDS, the affluent world would have to pay attention to the threat of a TB so difficult to treat, and to the dire but real possibility that "superbugs," strains resistant to every known antibiotic, would spread across borders—between homeless shelters and Park Avenue in New York, between poor and wealthy nations. "We've got to say, 'MDR is a threat to everyone,' " Jim declared. "We can scare the world, and if we do this project right, we can have a global impact."

"Okay," Paul said. "But let's try ten patients first."

===

They started treating patients late in August 1996, transporting Zanmi Lasante's TB program to Carabayllo, and tailoring it to MDR and other local circumstances. They already had an indigenous team: a group of young Peruvians trained as community health workers and Jaime to direct them. Farmer and Kim also imported a small crew from Boston: a brilliant epidemiologist named Meche Becerra, still in training at the Harvard School of Public Health, and two female students from Harvard Medical School, protégées of Farmer and Kim, who came virtually to live in Carabayllo, sleeping in one of the small rooms upstairs in the Father Jack Roussin Center. The medical students examined the patients and managed side effects, not as if they were real doctors yet but as Farmer's pupils. The entire medical team—the students, Jaime, a Peruvian doctor, several nurses, and Farmer— exchanged information by e-mail daily. Farmer sent orders in great detail and devised the drug regimens for every patient, inventing tricks, as he put it, for the most resistant cases. For a time, Jim did some doctoring himself, then turned exclusively to training and management and, later, attempts at fund-raising. They had many problems, especially at first. When, for instance, the health workers learned they'd be visiting the homes of MDR patients, they staged a small insurrection, demanding more pay. Jim and Jaime quelled it in a typical PIH way—Jim arranged a university scholarship for the ringleader, which took him away to Mexico. But the greatest difficulty, the only one they couldn't seem to solve, had to do with politics.

The Peruvian authorities didn't want to hear that their model TB program had a flaw, and it didn't help that Harvard doctors brought the news. Some of the authorities were downright hostile. *Médicos aventureros,* adventuring doctors, one Peruvian physician called Farmer and Kim. One said to Jaime, "Paul Farmer, he's a gringo. How could a gringo know about TB? There's no TB in the United States."

"He *looks* like a gringo," Jaime answered mildly. "But he's a fake gringo."

Neither Paul nor Jim had a license to practice in Peru. Early on, the TB director himself threatened to expel them—and he might have, if Jim and Paul and Jaime hadn't pleaded with a friend of the director's, a nun, to intercede on their behalf. But though they were allowed to continue, they had to get official permission to treat every MDR patient they found, and the authorities insisted that *las normas,* the norms of the national program, be strictly observed. All patients had to complete standard treatment and retreatment before their cases could be deemed "treatment failures." Only then could Socios take over.

Soon, these rules became excruciating. One of the young Harvard doctors—her name was Sonya Shin—had found a probable MDR victim in Carabayllo, a young man named David Carbajal, and though both she and Farmer had begged the authorities, they weren't allowed to treat him. So young Sonya had to watch him die. Afterward, she helped David's sister shave his face and clothe him for the funeral. Consoling Sonya, David's parents said, "It's a problem in the system. The system couldn't do another regimen, because of the fear they would be admitting a bigger problem." They understood the circumstances more clearly than Farmer, in his fury, could. He wrote an angry letter to the TB managers. This had no effect at all. Inappropriate behavior in a foreign doctor, they replied.

Jaime had already tried to reason with his countrymen, the Peruvian TB authorities, asking that they let Socios have patients earlier, at least once the first round of DOTS had failed and before patients went through the standard retreatment regimen. Socios would pay for everything, he had said. But the leaders of the program demurred. They didn't want to set a precedent, they explained. Though he didn't agree with them, Jaime understood their reasons.

Peru's TB program had come into being back in 1991 largely because of protests staged by residents of places like Carabayllo and by their nuns and priests. Some current leaders of the program had joined in the demonstrations. In an era of fiscal austerity in Peru, they had managed to get the government to put up the money for DOTS, and they had used it well. They had ended decades of improper treatment. A scandal about MDR now might threaten all their hard-won progress. But if they let Socios create a new standard for dealing with MDR around Carabayllo, they would have to meet that standard throughout the country. They didn't have the money to do that, not unless they took it from their DOTS program, and that would mean a return to the conditions that had spawned MDR here in the first place.

The Peruvians didn't have Paul's or Jim's freedom of action. It would only hurt their cause if they complained, for instance, that they could afford to treat all strains of TB for just a fraction of the money President Fujimori was spending on fighter jets. Besides, the Peruvians hadn't invented the *normas*. In January 1997, after David Carbajal had died, Jaime told Farmer, "If you want to change this, forget the national program. You have to go to higher authorities."

=====

Farmer agreed, and he thought he knew a suitable forum.

He'd been invited to give a speech about tuberculosis in Chicago at the end of February—at the annual North American meeting of an old and distinguished organization called the International Union Against Tuberculosis and Lung Disease. Officials from WHO's TB division would be on hand, along with many bureaucrats and public health specialists and medical school professors, all members of the confederacy of people who had made TB control the principal work of their lives. In Geneva once, I heard several of them refer to their tribe as "TB," in phrases such as "TB and HIV have to work together."

Farmer had some friends in "TB"—it was an old friend who had arranged this speaking engagement. But many members of "TB" had never heard of Farmer. Safe to say that many people at the lecture would know less about his ideas than he did about theirs.

Farmer knew that a lot of his audience didn't believe one should treat MDR in an impoverished locale: treatment was too expensive and difficult in such a setting, and treating it was probably unnecessary, because MDR wasn't as contagious or virulent as regular TB and would likely die out in the face of a good DOTS program. In other words, a lot of the audience would view what Socios was doing in Carabayllo as quixotic, even heretical. Farmer also knew that many members of "TB" would view him as a mere clinician, too interested in patients to see the big picture—to see that what was really important wasn't curing individuals but stopping the transmission of the disease. He rejected that idea utterly: paying attention to individual patients was a moral imperative; it was also essential to controlling TB in communities, as he'd proven in Cange. But he didn't want to rile up the audience too much. So he'd written what he called a "wimpy" talk. A few days before traveling to Chicago, he rewrote it.

The revised speech began temperately enough, but then Farmer intoned from the lectern, "Myths and mystifications about MDR-TB," and began reciting a rather long list. He read a quotation from WHO: "MDR-TB is too expensive to treat in poor countries; it detracts attention and resources from treating drug-susceptible disease." But was treating MDR-TB really too expensive? he asked. "Even if TB control is to be governed by considerations of cost-effectiveness, it should be easy to show that failure to diagnose and treat MDR-TB is what is really costly." The audience should consider the case of the family in Texas in which one member had exposed nine others to MDR. "Care for these ten persons alone exceeded one million dollars."

Myth number two: Some people thought that DOTS alone would stop outbreaks of MDR. This was nonsense, Farmer said. What would happen, he asked the audience, if programs treated drug-susceptible TB successfully and let MDR flourish? Transmission of MDR would continue, and even where MDR cases were now a tiny percentage of all TB cases, their relative importance would grow. Moreover, DOTS would amplify already existing drug resistance. In short, failure loomed for programs now deemed success stories.

What about the belief that MDR was less virulent and contagious than regular TB? Mere wishful thinking, Farmer said, moving on through his list of "myths and mystifications," through, that is, notions shared by many in "TB." He might as well have called half of his audience fools and villains.

"Thank you, Paul, for that provocative talk," said the moderator, a TB specialist from the U.S. Centers for Disease Control, a friend of Farmer's named Ken Castro.

Farmer was on his way offstage. He turned back. "Excuse me, Ken, but why do you qualify my talk as provocative? I just said we should treat sick people, if we have the technology."

In Lima a few days later, Jaime Bayona heard a rumor that someone in the audience had called the director of Peru's national TB program and told him, "Paul Farmer says you're killing patients." But at least his protest was lodged, and the higher authorities had noticed.

CHAPTER 17

Back in 1994 Ophelia had written, in a letter to Paul: "I am grateful to know about your budding relationship with Didi, and I am pleased for you, really I am."

The new woman in Farmer's life, Didi Bertrand, was the daughter of the schoolmaster in Cange, and "the most beautiful woman in Cange," people at Zanmi Lasante often said. Farmer had known her for a long time and had courted her for about two years when they got married—in Cange in 1996, in the midst of the hectic early phase of the project in Peru. Jim Kim and an old friend from Duke were Farmer's best men; Père Lafontant and three Catholic priests presided; about four thousand people came, including all of Cange. Somehow Farmer found time for the ceremonies, and for a second wedding reception back in Boston.

═══

By now Peru was taxing PIH's resources severely. On average, the drugs to treat just one patient cost between fifteen and twenty thousand dollars. And the number of patients kept growing. Already there were about fifty Carabayllanos in treatment. Their average age was twenty-nine. They were students, unemployed youths, housewives, street vendors, bus drivers, health workers. The actual numbers seemed small, but those fifty MDR cases represented about 10 percent of all active cases of TB in the slum, about ten times more than might have been expected. No telling how many others they had been infecting as they'd traveled around Lima, coughing. No telling either how many people in other parts of the city already had MDR, but Jaime was collecting reports of hundreds in other neighborhoods. In Carabayllo itself, the Socios workers found entire families sick and dying with what turned out to be genetically related strains of the disease—a phenomenon common enough that the health workers gave it a name, *familias tebeceanas,* tuberculosis families.

Ophelia worried. What had once looked like a manageable project seemed to be metastasizing. When Paul and Jim described the project as an AMC, she'd say, "That's fine, boys. I agree. But where's the dosh?"

At the Brigham, a friend of theirs named Howard Hiatt was asking himself much the same question. Hiatt was in his seventies and a personage in medicine—a former dean of the Harvard School of Public Health and former chief of medicine at Beth Israel Hospital, now a professor at Harvard Medical School. He was charged, among other duties, with lending advice and assistance to young doctors pursuing unconventional careers. Paul and Jim were among his favorites, and they were making him nervous. Where, he wondered, were they getting their second-line drugs? How in the world were they paying for them? Then one day the president of the Brigham stopped Hiatt in a corridor. "Your friends Farmer and Kim are in trouble with me. They owe this hospital ninety-two thousand dollars."

Hiatt looked into the matter. "Sure enough. Paul and Jim would stop at the Brigham pharmacy before they left for Peru and fill their briefcases with drugs. They had sweet-talked various people into letting them walk away with the drugs." He was amused, all in all. "That's their Robin Hood attitude."

In fact, they'd only borrowed the drugs. Tom White soon sent the Brigham a check for the entire bill, along with a note saying he thought the hospital ought to be more generous toward the poor.

"Better to ask forgiveness than permission." That had been Father Jack's favorite saying. It was Farmer's rule of thumb. When he and Jim had first resolved to take on Carabayllo's epidemic, he had gone to Tom White and said, "Just buy the drugs for ten patients. We promise there won't be more." Even then Farmer had known this was what he called "a fib." He had come back many times since to ask White for more money. White shared in the general nervousness. He wanted to leave this life without a nickel, he often said. As the number of patients grew, he began to wonder if Paul and Jim would upset his calculations. "For a while there, I thought they'd spend all my money before I died." But he never turned them down.

To many seasoned managers of public health projects, what Farmer and Kim were doing would have looked quite reckless—like a stunt, as some would later insinuate. They didn't have a guaranteed supply of drugs, only the determination to obtain the drugs and the charm to get away with borrowing. They were borrowing their laboratory services, too, from Massachusetts. They lacked proper institutional support. The weight of expert opinion stood against them. Their organization was small and it had other projects, in Haiti and Boston and elsewhere, and Peru put a strain on everyone.

Jim had to travel to Carabayllo at least once a month. Farmer had to go there slightly more often. He didn't put much work aside for Peru, not his duties in Haiti or his service at the Brigham or his teaching at Harvard or his growing number of speaking engagements. He just added Peru to his itinerary.

Often he'd make two-day trips. He'd leave Cange before dawn and drive to Port-au-Prince. Sometimes he'd get stuck in traffic and, turning the truck over to a Haitian assistant, climb out and jog the last half mile to the airport. He'd catch the early flight to Miami, then fly on to Lima, arriving in Carabayllo late the same night. Starting early the next morning, he'd stride up and down the dusty hills with the Harvard student doctors or with one of the Socios nurses, visiting patients in their shacks. Later, when the local TB authorities had warmed up a bit to Socios, the patients were brought to the Jack Roussin Center, and he saw them there in a small room with a table and a concrete floor. That way he could see a larger number. He'd work until it was time to leave for the airport. He'd take the night flight to Miami, catch the early morning plane to Port-au-Prince, and arrive back in Cange by afternoon. He spent about twenty-two of the forty-eight hours just traveling, longer if flights got delayed or canceled, or Zanmi Lasante's truck broke down, or an accident blocked the stretch of Highway 3 up Morne Kabrit, or rain had made the streams that crossed that road impassable.

Farmer hadn't been feeling well when he gave his speech in Chicago, in February 1997. He felt worse when he got to Boston to spend a month of service at the Brigham. "I must be exhausted," he remembered thinking. "Everyone told me something like this would happen." He prided himself on being a fast diagnostician, but he took his time on his own case. He kept on working, and his symptoms got worse. He reviewed them: nausea, vomiting, fatigue, night sweats. "Oh, my God," he thought. "I've got MDR."

His wife, Didi, had begun her studies in Paris. So for now, when he was in Boston, Farmer still camped in the basement of the PIH building—PIH-ers called it "the cave." He woke up there in the middle of the night bathed in sweat, thinking, "If I do have MDR, I've exposed all my patients to it."

He went to a radiologist friend, swore him to secrecy, and had his chest X-rayed. He studied the film. It was normal.

He called Didi in Paris at least once a day. She told him over the phone, *"You must go to a doctor."*

"Look, I *am* a doctor. Let me finish the month at the Brigham and go to Haiti. Then I'll rest."

He finally made the diagnosis on the morning of his last day of Brigham service. The night before, he'd turned down pizza, and that morning the smell of coffee nauseated him. Classic for hepatitis, he thought. Revulsion at foods you love. In the bathroom he saw that his urine was dark. "Oh, no. I do have hepatitis. Which kind? B? No, I've been vaccinated. Not C. I don't do drugs. A? But how?" He'd discovered ceviche in Lima. Perhaps he had eaten some tainted fish.

When he got to the Brigham, he stopped at the lab and asked them to do tests on him at once. He stayed around to see the first result, his red blood count. "It's way out of whack," he thought. He felt dehydrated, so while the other lab results were still pending, he called Jim Kim on the house phone. Jim was back in Boston, too, managing a floor at the Brigham. "Jim, I'm coming up to your unit. I need fluids." Then Farmer lay down in his suit in one of the rooms on Jim's floor, feeling rather cheerful. After the IV nurse rehydrated him, he got off the bed and joined the infectious disease specialist he was training, a young woman. "Marla," he told her, "I feel worse. Let's do rounds early."

Marla was usually impatient with him. She'd interrupt his constant in-hospital socializing, saying, "Farmer, shut up. Let's get working." Now she said, "You're psycho. Let someone take over for you."

"Marla, I finish today."

She went away scowling. He went into a patient's room, and was in the midst of diagnosing a case of acute prostatitis—it was obvious— when Marla returned. Her face looked blanched, he thought. "Paul, your liver functions are so high the machine couldn't do them. They had to dilute it."

"All right. I give up." He went back to the room in Jim's unit, got into a johnny, and surrendered himself to illness.

Hepatitis A is only rarely fatal, but his case was severe—Jim and some other doctors worried that he might need a liver transplant. Farmer was so sick for a time that he could hardly make his voice audible. Nevertheless, a few nights after he took to his hospital bed a young PIH-er got a call from him, a tiny, squeaky voice issuing instructions about drug procurement for Peru. When he got out of the hospital two weeks later, Ophelia sent him and Didi to a hotel in southern France, Paul's first real vacation in years. Nine months later he had a daughter, named Catherine. So everything turned out all right.

But hearing him tell the story, I wondered at his recklessness. At the Brigham he'd been preaching the importance of hepatitis A vaccination, especially for middle-aged people. He told me, "I was embarrassed." But only, it seemed, for failing to get the shot, not for ignoring his symptoms during an entire month. He hadn't told Ophelia or his mother he was sick, and I wondered if that was because he knew they would try to make him stop working. Doctors are notorious for taking peculiar views of their own bodies. They tend to develop hypochondria in medical school and, once they get over it, if they do, tend to think they're invulnerable. Many people refuse to set their work aside for matters of personal convenience. But Farmer seemed to be unwilling to set it aside for any reason. It was as if he couldn't allow himself to be the one to set it aside. A force stronger than his own will had to intervene, like the car that had hit him back in 1988.

Speaking of his bout of hepatitis, Farmer told me, "If I get sick, it'll be *nearly* fatal." He was drawing a contrast between himself and the world's poor. A generous thought, but his habit of disregarding his health hardly seemed like a way of expressing "pragmatic solidarity." Given the responsibilities for other lives he'd taken on, it seemed to me he'd done the opposite.

On the other hand, at some point—I'm not sure exactly when—I realized that I'd become inclined to hold Farmer to a higher standard than I did most people, including myself. And, as a rule, to see him in action was to excuse him.

═

The MDR project was making progress with patients, and the Peruvian TB doctors had noticed. Accordingly, Farmer and Kim were making progress with them.

One day, when it was clear that the project was succeeding, I followed Farmer to an appointment at the Children's Hospital in downtown Lima. When he emerged from the noisy, smoky traffic jam in front of the hospital, a small entourage of Peruvian medical people rushed out to claim him, then hurried him past the men hawking toilet paper and balloons and newspapers, then past the armed guard at the front door. Farmer was, I figured from the fuss, *médico aventurero* no more around here. He looked worried, though. Or maybe I only imagined this, thinking he ought to be. He and Jim and Jaime had tried hard to establish collegial relations with the Peruvian medical establishment, and now, because of traffic, he'd kept a group of proud doctors waiting over an hour for him.

Farmer pulled a stethoscope out of the pocket of his rumpled black suit jacket and draped it over his neck as we entered a maze of narrow, concrete-walled corridors—the hospital's tuberculosis wing. He was walking fast. Then, all of a sudden, he stopped.

A family of three stood in the hallway up ahead. A little boy and his mother and father. The mother was slender and wore a skirt and a T-shirt with a picture of Mickey Mouse on the front. She hung back, half-hidden around a corner, while the father came forward. Farmer and the father opened their arms simultaneously and bear-hugged each other. ("In my culture we don't shake hands," Farmer was always telling me, trying to reform me in this way, too, I'd begun to feel.) Hurriedly, he asked for news of the child.

The little boy was chubby, obviously healthy. He stood close to his father. When Farmer crouched down and held out his arms, the child came forward on his own stubby legs, in a rolling, waddling gait, giggling as he advanced headlong toward Farmer, then turning around and waddling back toward his father. A happy-looking dance. "Christian! Look at you!" cried Farmer. His face had turned bright red. He wore the wild-looking grin with which he greeted old friends. He turned to me. "This was a terrible case," he said in a low voice, in English.

Nearly two years ago, a doctor from this hospital had called Jaime Bayona at Socios headquarters and said, "We have a child here you have to help us with." By the time of that phone call, Christian had been lying in bed for months. Jen Furin, the Harvard medical student who worked with Sonya in Carabayllo, went to the hospital. The child she found there was three years old and weighed only about twenty-two pounds. He labored to breathe, and the oxygen mask had made sores around his nose. Tuberculosis had invaded both his lungs, it had begun eating his spine, and it had fractured the long bones of his legs. He had gone through the six months of standard short-course chemotherapy. Then the lab had cultured his TB and found it resistant to several drugs. Christian was being given those same drugs when Jen arrived. The doctors were obeying las normas, applying the WHO retreatment plan.

Jen had done most of the actual doctoring. Farmer had devised the regimen for Christian. He'd talked about the case to both Peruvian and American TB experts, but no one in the world knew much about treating children with second-line drugs. "Here was the received wisdom. You can't use fluoroquinolones or ethambutol at high doses in kids. Where did this come from? Fluoroquinolones cause cartilage damage in immature beagle pups. High-dose ethambutol is associated with optic neuritis and loss of color vision in a small proportion of adults, but kids can't report loss of color vision, so it shouldn't be used. This was a big part of the discussion, and here was a child literally wasting away, his flesh and bones consumed by MDR, in front of our eyes."

Farmer proposed an "empiric" regimen—a regimen based on his best guesses—which consisted of high-dose ethambutol and four second-line drugs, including a fluoroquinolone. To get official approval, he told the Peruvian doctors that he'd discussed the matter with every world-renowned expert, and studied the pediatric literature. This was true. He didn't say that the pediatric literature contained nothing at all about treating MDR. "It was a matter of merely applying infectious disease knowledge," he would tell me. He based the dosing on the drug manufacturers' recommendations, which had nothing to say about children but advised the use of so many milligrams of drug per so many kilograms of body weight. He'd often done this with other pediatric illnesses in Haiti. He recommended a very aggressive course of second-line drugs for Christian. Too aggressive, said some of the American doctors he consulted. "Who, I might add, had never treated a baby with MDR." The Peruvians had no experience with such cases either. They accepted Farmer's recommendation. The child was clearly dying, and in agony. So why not try it?

Farmer had learned, through e-mail, that Christian was coming along well, but he hadn't known how well until this moment in the hall at the Children's Hospital. The child could actually run! Farmer grinned, and a blush spread from his high forehead and over his neck and, I imagined, down past his necktie toward his feet, as the child waddled around giggling in front of him and the father beamed down at the child and the mother peered out from around the corner, smiling, too.

Then it was over. Christian's wasn't the main case Farmer had been asked to consult on today. He was making this hospital visit on Jaime Bayona's instructions, as a favor to a Peruvian TB doctor whose own daughter was sick. Farmer's escorts shepherded him into an office—a whitewashed ceiling, concrete walls, a team of doctors, and a little girl in a dress. A string of X rays and CT films were mounted in a viewer along one wall, pictures of the interior of the little girl's chest. Farmer made apologies for his lateness to the doctors, bowing a little at the waist, and then turned with them to the films. The little girl had pulmonary TB. "Infiltrates. Not good," Farmer said in Spanish to the doctors.

He studied the report from the Massachusetts State Lab. It was unequivocal. I looked over his shoulder at the sheet of paper—a list of the five first-line antibiotics with the letter R for "resistant" next to each one. The child, the doctor's daughter, had gone through DOTS and was now several months into the retreatment regimen. That is, she was being treated with all five of those same drugs.

"This is terrible," Farmer murmured to me in English, from the side of his mouth.

He knelt down and listened through his stethoscope to the girl's lungs. Then, smiling, he looked up at her father and said, "She has asthma. Just like me. She's adorable, like my Catherine." Then Farmer stood and began a long spiel in Spanish, directed to the little girl's father and the other doctors. "I do not know more than this medical team, my esteemed colleagues here. She has wheezing and a worsening CT scan since February. It's worrisome." He reviewed the options. They could perform a new laboratory analysis, on the chance that the Massachusetts State Lab had made a mistake, even though it had a nearly flawless record, well-certified. Or they could wait and monitor the child's condition, even though it was getting worse. *Or* they could trust the lab work, abandon the DOTS retreatment regimen, and begin giving her Farmer's own favorite pediatric regimen of second-line drugs. He preferred this last course, he said. "This is my prejudice."

He smiled some more at the doctors. "As you know, from our experience together, working shoulder to shoulder."

The room seemed full of strong feeling, covered with professional courtesy. The little girl's father stood behind his daughter. He maintained a smile throughout. He kept his shoulders erect. He was trying hard, it seemed to me, to hold on to his professional composure. He was a TB doctor after all. But when Farmer spoke to him about his daughter, the man reached out to touch her shoulders, and he seemed to hold his breath. "He knew," Jaime Bayona would tell me later. "He *knew* for months that she had MDR." But the man hadn't dared go against the national program's strict *normas*. One could imagine his reasons. He would have been risking his job, and jobs like his were hard enough to come by in Peru that to risk it would be to risk the survival of his entire family. Jaime had taken matters into his own hands. He'd had the girl's sputum sent to Boston, circumventing the national lab, and when the results had come back, her father, an old friend, had begged Jaime—*begged,* Jaime insisted—that Farmer examine her. Because Farmer's opinions had weight now with a lot of Peruvian doctors.

The father had known beforehand that Farmer would prescribe second-line therapy and so had the assembled doctors. ("They were just waiting for Paul to pronounce," Jaime would say later on. Indeed, soon afterward the doctors would place the girl on Farmer's regimen, and she would begin to recover, suffering few side effects.) So the consult was really just a charade. Farmer played out the rest of his part with aplomb. He promised to send his report and recommendations to the father by e-mail. He ticked off the reasons for optimism on his fingers. "It is possible she may still have rifabutin on her side. She's in good shape. She has only a little lung damage. Her resistance isn't total. We are ready to help you in any way that we can."

Soon, with many thank-yous and bowings and scrapings and warmest wishes to their beautiful wives and distinguished husbands, Farmer departed.

On the way out of the hospital he said, speaking of the little girl, "The child is wheezing and has a worsening CT. She's on all five first-

line drugs and she's resistant to all of them. And I had to say, 'I wonder why she isn't getting better,' and go through the pathophysiology.
Instead of saying, 'What's the matter with you people?' They don't
want to believe in MDR. The delicate thing is, you want to make
progress with them. Insult them and forget it. They want to do the
right thing. They're just following instructions from on high."

But Christian, the little boy in the hall, made an eloquent argument for adding flexibility to the *normas*. "A couple more cases like
Christian's and they'll come around," Farmer was saying as we walked
across the parking lot toward the Socios car. Then, turning to open his
door, Farmer saw Christian's mother, the woman in the Mickey
Mouse shirt. She had followed him at a distance. Now she approached,
lowered her eyes, and said in Spanish, "I want to say many thanks."

Farmer looked away, just a quick glance to left and right. I'd seen
him do this in patients' rooms at the Brigham—look at the patient,
then glance up at the TV for a moment, then return, as if disconnect-
ing so as to reconnect fully. He gazed at the woman and pursed his lips
and said softly in Spanish, "For me, it is a privilege."

CHAPTER 18

In April 1998 a special meeting of "TB" was convened at the American Academy of Arts and Sciences in Boston, a meeting to present early results from the small MDR-treatment project in Peru. The meeting was Howard Hiatt's idea.

Socios was now treating more than one hundred people with MDR in the northern slums of Lima. They had been treating the first fifty-three for the better part of two years, and the results were in. It appeared that more than 85 percent were cured. Their patients were younger on average and had fewer accompanying illnesses than Dr. Iseman's in Denver, and as with many diseases, youthfulness and the absence of comorbidity were therapeutic advantages. Even so, the cure rate was remarkable. "An astonishing result," Howard Hiatt had said. The world must hear this news, he'd declared. He hoped, among other things, that if the right people heard it, PIH might be able to secure new financing for their project.

A lot of the world's ranking tuberculosis experts had agreed to come to the meeting, including Arata Kochi, the head of WHO's TB program. Farmer had cultivated him. Equally important, Kochi had been a student of Hiatt's at the Harvard School of Public Health.

Kochi had labored for years to sell DOTS to the world, and as I understood his motives, he felt he had to quell the bad publicity Farmer had begun stirring up. Before the meeting he had decided that WHO should probably have a strategy that included MDR treatment in places where there was significant drug resistance. One of his staff had come up with a new, catchy term, "DOTS-plus."

Some years after the event, Arata Kochi told me, in his clipped English (Japanese is his native tongue): "MDR is basically because of human errors. If you can't treat it right, don't do it. Secondly, many country can't afford. Difficult, expensive. And of course we use MDR as kind of a scare tactics. But in program review in South Africa we found thirty-four percent of whole TB budget for a few cases of MDR, and they had a lousy DOTS program. We said, Use your money for DOTS. Then Paul Farmer came. A very different approach. Similar to HIV activists. All good clinicians without significant public health experience. Patient in front of me is the most important thing. An unsolvable conflict. They are very articulate and issue is very emotional. How to react? Tremendous challenge for me. These guys, they are screaming. They want to shoot us. Politically we have to respond. Positively. Same time we have to start dialogue."

Kochi used the term *DOTS-plus* in his opening remarks at the meeting. "That's brilliant! That's great!" Jim Kim told him later, over cocktails. So Farmer and Kim got some of what they hoped for from "TB" before the meeting even started. Speaking about all this some years later, Kochi smiled and said, "DOTS-plus. The world is changing. We have to change, too. If you cannot beat them, join them." He added, "Then, to some extent, we can control them."

=

Kochi had made a strategic concession. In effect, he'd made MDR treatment discussable. But the discussion itself was just beginning.

When panels on international health gather, whether in Switzerland, Indonesia, or Boston, they occupy one place and atmosphere. A room with a huge table or many tables made into a giant rectangle, bottled water and name cards at each seat. Over the rattle of coffee cups, to the shuffle and click of the slide projector, the experts read their prepared remarks, technical terms and acronyms abounding, now and then old saws—"Don't let perfect be the enemy of good." In the corridors and hallways outside the lecture rooms, you might, for instance, hear an Italian TB expert say of a Canadian one, "I am going to physically aggress him!" But inside the rooms, calm usually prevails. It's easy to drift away on the voices, imagining colors in the accents—pinks and purples from the Caribbean and the Indian subcontinent, black and white from Japan—and forget that what is really going on is the writing of prescriptions that may affect the lives of billions.

Hiatt presided, tall and thin, uttering the opening remarks at his usual deliberate pace, as if his tongue weighed every word. The atmosphere was civil, but there were a few heated discussions on scientific issues. An argument of a different sort began on the afternoon of the first day of the meeting, when a bearded man named Alex Goldfarb leaned over his microphone and said, in sonorously accented English, "So. Russia is a TB nightmare."

Goldfarb was a rumpled-looking microbiologist, a former refusenik in the latter days of the Soviet Union. He was working now for the Soros Foundation on the TB epidemic in Russia. One hundred thousand of that country's prison inmates had active TB, Goldfarb said, and most if not all were being treated with the worst possible regimen—with a single drug—because the government hadn't come up with the money to buy more. "So. It is a nightmare. So most of these one hundred thousand inmates will probably die without ever knowing whether they have MDR-TB or not." His group was trying to sort things out and "eemplement some sort of rational approach." They were setting up demonstration projects, DOTS projects, in several places. There was no telling yet how many Russians had MDR, but it was certain the percentage in the prisons was high.

"Now what to do with these cases?" Goldfarb asked. He answered, "I do not have the slightest idea." He turned to Farmer. "And I would very much like to know, how much drugs did you use for your fifty-three cases and how much did they cost? We can probably *try* to eemplement MDR treatment, at least in prison. I don't think it can be done in the community in Russia, but in prison, at least, if there is money. But the question is the cost."

Farmer mustered the best case he could, but in the end he had to name the real figures. "I'm not saying that it's not expensive. It's been very costly. I'm not saying that it's not going to be difficult. But I will say, as Dr. Bayona has suggested, that we have managed to overcome those obstacles for that small number of patients. And that leads me to believe that it would be possible ultimately . . ."

A PIH ally raised her hand. Costs would only rise if the world delayed in taking on MDR, she said. But another expert said, "I'm not sure that no matter how compelling a case that this group or any other group makes, there's going to be all of a sudden an outpouring of money to treat." Others raised their voices. Another PIH ally declared, "I don't think this is a conference of donors, so I don't think we should be expected to come out of this with pledges, but to say that this is something that the world should pay attention to. I remember signing the oath to assist the patient and do him no harm. I don't really remember signing that I would do it in a cost-effective way." There was scattered applause from the young PIH-ers in the room.

Then Goldfarb spoke up again, his voice calm and acidic. "I want to share with you a simple reality. I have six million dollars. With three million dollars I can eemplement DOTS for five thousand Russian prison inmates. And assuming that ten percent have MDR-TB, forty-five hundred will be cured and five hundred will go down with MDR-TB and die. And there's nothing much you can do. So. I have a choice. And my choice is to use another three million dollars to treat the five hundred with MDR-TB, or go to another region and treat another five thousand. I'm working with leemited resources. So my choice is not involved in the human rights of five hundred people, but five hundred people versus five thousand people. And this is a very practical question for me, because I have six million dollars. And the second question is that if I disclose to the Russian people that I spent six thousand dollars per case in MDR-TB in the prisons with tens of thousands of people dying all around, they will tell me that I am building a golden palace for a selected few. So for those of us who *have* to make those decisions with leemited resources, it's a very serious question."

There was consternation in the room. Hiatt had to bang the gavel. He asked Goldfarb if he couldn't see his way to using some of Soros's money, in a pilot project perhaps, to address the question of how MDR affected DOTS.

"Well, I'm sorry," Goldfarb retorted. "I have to comment. When we talk about Mr. Kochi, who's not doing an experiment but whose job is to try to control TB globally, there is a different set of priorities. I can't afford doing a pilot project. We're not doing a pilot project."

"My understanding," said Hiatt pleasantly, "is that my former student, Dr. Kochi, is thinking about control of tuberculosis, not just in 1998 and '99, because he recognizes that he's not going to control the problem worldwide, but is thinking about controlling the problem over the next decade, or decades."

The young PIH-ers glared at Goldfarb. But he'd made an argument that they'd have to answer, sooner or later.

=

Jim Kim tried rhetoric first in the opening speech the next day. Many people had asked him, he told the crowd, why a little organization like PIH had taken on such a costly and difficult task in Peru. They were right to wonder. "We actually had to make a choice that we would not feed four thousand more children in Haiti perhaps. And if any of you have been to Haiti, there's hardly anything more morally compelling than the situation of landless peasants in the central plateau."

But, Jim went on, they'd had "a dream": "the dream that someday we might sit in this room." That there might be "a TB All-Star Weekend." He said, "We took on this project because we thought that by proving that one could do community-based treatment of multidrug-resistant TB, that we might have the opportunity to work with a roomful of people like you. To actually *expand* resources to a problem that afflicts the populations we serve."

Other speakers had talked about the need to generate "political will" for treating TB, as if each country had to solve its own problem. But, Jim said, political will was hardly the issue in a place such as Zaire, whose most recent president had stolen about 30 percent of the money loaned by foreign governments and the World Bank. For places like Zaire, money to deal with TB and MDR-TB would have to come from elsewhere. "There are more billionaires today than ever before," Jim declared. "We are talking about wealth that we've never seen before. And the only time that I hear talk of shrinking resources among people like us, among academics, is when we talk about things that have to do with poor people." The PIH project in Peru could be replicated, and some of what was needed were endorsements from "academics with clout" and the support of "the TB community."

Jim said, "And let me just conclude this, my brief remarks here at this TB All-Star Weekend, by paraphrasing someone of our tribe, of Paul's tribe and my tribe of anthropologists. Margaret Mead once said, Never underestimate the ability of a small group of committed individuals to change the world." He paused. "Indeed, they are the only ones who ever have."

CHAPTER 19

Many of the policy makers in TB control had now heard the case—the fine clinical results from Peru, and epidemiological evidence that DOTS would fail in a setting of substantial drug resistance. The meeting had also produced—of course—a committee to study the feasibility of DOTS-plus programs. But the arguments about treating MDR were far from over.

In international health near the turn of the twenty-first century, a mentality nearly opposite to Jim Kim's optimism prevailed. It borrowed from the nineteenth-century utilitarian philosophers, from the notion that one should provide the greatest good for the greatest number, and it was expressed in a language of realism. The world had limited resources. Nations whose resources weren't just limited but scarce had to make the best possible uses of the little they had. Other countries and international institutions might help out, but these days, if you wanted money from big donors for health projects in poor countries, if you wanted to be taken seriously, your proposals had to pass a test, called cost-effectiveness analysis.

The general technique was used first in engineering, later on in war and medicine. You calculated the cost of a public health project or medical procedure and tried to quantify its effectiveness. Then you compared the results for competing projects or procedures. Farmer and Kim made similar calculations when trying to decide what to do next in Cange. But it seemed to them that the high councils in international health often used this analytic tool to rationalize an irrational status quo: MDR treatment was cost-effective in a place like New York, but not in a place like Peru.

By the time of the meeting in Boston, the project in Peru had begun to establish a new paradigm. It was a challenge to the uses of cost-effectiveness analysis not only philosophically but also factually. The World Health Organization had declared MDR treatment largely ineffective, but not on the basis of any substantial trials. Now Kim and Farmer and Jaime Bayona and the others in Socios had proven that effective treatment was possible, even in a slum in a relatively poor country. Experts in TB control had declared MDR treatment inordinately costly, but no one had tried to reduce the main expense, which was high-priced drugs. Shortly after the Boston meeting, Jim Kim went to WHO headquarters in Geneva. No one he talked to there even knew that the patents on all but one class of the second-line antibiotics had expired years ago. And no one there seemed very interested when he declared, "We can drive down the prices by ninety to ninety-five percent."

Jim didn't know exactly how to make that happen. Make the assertion, then figure out the means—this was his strategy. "The big-shot strategy," Farmer called it, approvingly.

≡

Jim was born in South Korea and grew up in Muscatine, Iowa, in the 1970s. For as long as he could remember, the place had seemed too small for his ambitions. He hardly noticed the Mississippi flowing by the lovely old downtown or the fragrances of grains on summer nights or even the famous local produce, the Muscatine melon. He detasseled corn only once. But, like every schoolboy in town, he knew Mark Twain had praised Muscatine for its sunsets—and didn't know for decades that Twain had said this only to make a joke about his sleeping habits: "The sunrises are also said to be exceedingly fine. I do not know."

Jim's father had schemed and charmed his way out of North Korea and become, proudly, Muscatine's periodontist, with an office upstairs on Main Street. Jim's mother had come from South Korea—a grandfather had served as a minister to the last Korean king—and she had studied at Union Theological Seminary with Reinhold Niebuhr and Paul Tillich and become a Confucian scholar, and ended up for many years a housewife in Muscatine. A small, elegant woman walking across the local golf course when her children were too young to play alone, diligently trying to make sense of American sports so she could understand her children's milieu. At every opportunity she took Jim and his siblings to Des Moines and Chicago so they'd know the world was larger than it seemed from Muscatine. She taught her three children, by example, the arts of debate around the kitchen table, while her husband, who had early morning appointments, went to bed grumbling that he didn't know what they had to talk about that was more important than a good night's sleep. She'd tell them to live "as if for eternity" and tutor them on current events, translating for Jim the images of famine and war that upset him on the TV news. Early on, Jim imagined himself becoming a doctor to treat such suffering, and excelling in science quickened his interest.

He was quarterback on the Muscatine High football team, a starting guard in basketball, the president of his class and its valedictorian. But the Kims were the only Asian family in town, except for the one that owned the Chinese restaurant. When they went to the malls of Iowa, adults stared and children followed them around, the bolder ones approaching, crying out, "Kiai!" and making as if to deliver karate chops. For Jim, embarrassment at his parents' Koreanness was the loneliest feeling of all. "Go, Hawkeye!" his father, booster of all things Iowan, would cry, Koreanizing the cheer for the University of Iowa's sports teams. Jim would correct him: "No, Dad. It's Hawk*eyes*."

He went to the University of Iowa and felt liberated there until he was told that Ivy League schools were better. He transferred to Brown, where he discovered an organization called the Third World Center. He became its director. He broke up with his Irish Catholic girlfriend because he suddenly believed he shouldn't date white women. He made his friends among black, Hispanic, and Asian students. He learned "the pimp walk." On parents' weekend he and his friends would dress up in black and stride around the campus, a phalanx of about thirty African

American and Hispanic students, and one Korean, sometimes chanting, sometimes maintaining a threatening silence, and noting with pleasure the double takes and frightened looks on the faces of some of the parents.

Before Brown, Jim hadn't known that the United States interned Japanese Americans during World War II. He read up on the subject, then lectured about it. He embraced the idea of Asian "racial solidarity." He didn't realize back then just how complex a matter this could be. He didn't find out until much later that, for example, Koreans were supposed to hate the Japanese. From time to time, doubts cropped up. It seemed as if, for other Asians at Brown, racial identity meant little more than eating with chopsticks and finding an Asian mate, and the paramount political issue seemed to be the "glass ceiling," the fact that Asians weren't yet rising to the very tops of institutions. But the idea of being a member of an oppressed minority was very alluring. Jim decided to learn his native language. "I wanted to learn Korean, be down with my people, be an authorized third world person, so I could say shit." He got a fellowship to travel to Seoul and happened on an interesting story for his Ph.D. thesis in anthropology—it had to do with the Korean pharmaceutical industry. In Seoul he did his research and made a mighty effort to fit in, hanging out at bars with new Korean friends and performing karaoke—beforehand on each occasion, he'd go to the bathroom and study the words to songs like "My Way."

He had left Iowa prepared, naturally enough, to think that ethnicity was the central problem of his life. By the time he came back from Korea to Harvard, to continue medical school and write his thesis, he had grown bored and a little disgusted with what was known in academic circles as the politics of racial identity. It seemed like an exercise in selfishness. "I discovered South Korea was doing just fine, and that what Koreans wanted was for me to write grant proposals so they could come to the States and get degrees. I had looked at student movements. They were all about Korean nationalism, just sort of troublemaking." When he met Farmer, he was ready to change directions. At one point during their talks in the old, one-room PIH office,

Farmer told him, "If you come to Haiti, I'll show you you're *blan,* as white as any white man." Jim thought of his black, Hispanic, and Asian friends at Brown, and how angry that remark would have made them.

He told Farmer that he felt liberated from "the self-hatred and evasion of ethnicity" he'd felt in Muscatine.

"It's good to have to come to understandings of that, but you've got to put that behind you now," said Farmer. "So what are you going to do? Be the first Asian to do some stupid thing like walk on the moon?"

They hadn't talked long before Jim declared that he wanted to make Farmer's preferential option for the poor his own life's work.

All his life, it seemed, Jim had been jumping at the next new thing, the bigger and better thing. Perhaps this was the residue of growing up in Muscatine with a cosmopolitan mother. "You're not Korean, you're *careen,*" Ophelia told him once. Jim himself said, "I tend to feel a problem's solved once I've thought it through." Then again, he was fond of overstatement, even when talking about himself. After all, he'd stuck with PIH for a decade by now, and done a lot of its most menial chores along the way. What Jim had, above all, was enthusiasm. He'd weigh facts against possibilities as if the two were equivalent. A lot of students had joined PIH after hearing him talk. Change the world? Of course they could. He really believed this, and he really believed that "a small group of committed individuals" could do it. He liked to say of PIH, "People think we're unrealistic. They don't know we're crazy."

═══

From his research in Korea, Jim already knew that the price of a drug may have little to do with its usefulness or the costs of manufacturing and distributing it. Often, the price is high because only one company makes it. A firm can secure this monopoly power through patents, but that wasn't the case with the second-line TB drugs. In the world, perhaps as many as 750,000 people suffered from MDR. Treating all of them would require a large quantity of drugs, because treatment lasted so long. So the potential market was big, but most people with the disease were poor, so actual demand was small. Not many companies made the drugs. Those that did could pretty much name their price.

Eli Lilly and the second-line drug capreomycin, for instance. After long badgering from Farmer, that company was finally selling PIH capreo in Peru—for $21.00 a vial. Farmer and Kim had bought the same drug, made by Lilly, for $29.90 a vial at the Brigham in Boston. Then they had discovered that it cost only $8.80 in Paris. So they'd tried to buy capreo in Paris but were told they couldn't. "There's a global shortage of capreo," the drug agent in Paris had told Farmer over the phone.

"Why?" Farmer asked.

"There seems to be an emergency."

"Where?"

"In Peru."

Jim went to Howard Hiatt and told him the story. "Looks like price gouging to me," Hiatt said. In fact, so-called differential pricing was standard in the world of large drug companies; Americans paid far more for their products than any other nationality. But Hiatt thought Lilly might want to pick up some good publicity by donating drugs to the project in Peru. He knew a member of Lilly's board. He and Jim went to work on the company, and meanwhile Jim began pursuing other angles.

Jim got WHO to agree to hold a meeting to encourage drug companies to produce more second-line antibiotics—he hoped to create competition, which would drive down prices. Then WHO backed out, and Jim convened the meeting himself in Boston. He wasn't above hyperbole or dramatics. At one moment he put a list of numbers up on the slide projector, describing very large potential demand for the second-line antibiotics, in order to impress the drug companies. The numbers themselves were accurate, but the demand they described wasn't real, because no one contemplating MDR treatment programs had the cash to buy the drugs. The tactic didn't work quite as Jim planned. Out in the audience there was a Dutchman in his twenties named Guido Bakker. He worked for a nonprofit company, the International Dispensary Association—IDA. It specialized in driving down the prices of essential drugs, the kinds of drugs that poor countries need most urgently. Bakker saw right through Jim's ploy. But he felt angry at the representatives from the for-profit drug companies. They started arguing that the prices for second-line TB drugs *ought* to remain high. Finally, Bakker announced from his seat, "IDA is going to do everything we can to lower prices, by exploring generic manufacturers."

The Dutch group's strategy was to ignore the giant multinational drug companies, the ones that mainly rely on research and brand names and patent protection, and to deal instead with the myriad smaller companies that make and sell, at greatly reduced prices, already invented generic drugs under different names (as acetaminophen instead of Tylenol in the United States, for instance). This seemed to Jim like a better idea than his own. His fondness for the new and better idea might be his salient weakness, but it sometimes served him well. He didn't care where an idea came from. He was forever reading books about corporate management, looking for tips from capitalists. He embraced Guido Bakker's plan. Ultimately, IDA and the renowned organization Doctors Without Borders took on the job of finding generic manufacturers of second-line drugs. IDA even talked some companies into making the drugs, and they assumed responsibility for quality control and distribution. And Doctors Without Borders put up the cash to buy the first shipments.

But other steps came first. Jim's task was like a logician's conundrum. To lower the prices of the drugs, he had to show that a lot of TB projects would use them. For a lot of projects to use them, the prices had to be lower. For the prices to be lower, the generic manufacturers would have to get involved. They'd be more inclined to get involved if WHO would put the second-line antibiotics on its official list of essential drugs. But rarely used drugs are by definition not essential. To break through this circular chain, Jim began to lobby WHO for the drugs' inclusion on the list.

The World Health Organization serves as the coordinating body for virtually all the world's ministries of health. It sets guidelines and standards, publishes recommended approaches, acts as an advisory group. It's where all the information about health and a lot of the complaints go, and it performs some crucial functions well, such as the collection and dissemination of worldwide epidemiological data. But it is perennially short of money, and like most parts of the United Nations it is infamously, inevitably, tangled in bureaucracy. It has a tendency to freeze in the face of controversy. The organization's critics said it had two mottoes: "Slow down" and "It's not our fault." Even Jim's strongest ally there got frightened when various eminent TB experts wrote to Geneva saying they couldn't countenance the elevation of second-line antibiotics to the essential drugs list. Some wrote that the plan wouldn't work. Others believed that if it did and prices fell, the drugs would become *too* widely available.

This worry had substance. In the real world, many places lacked even rudimentary health services, and others had clinics and hospitals staffed by the ignorant, the careless, the lazy. In the real world, some doctors and nurses peddled drugs on black markets, desperate patients sold their antibiotics to buy food, and stupid pharmacists mixed first-line TB drugs with cough medicine. Start distributing the second-line, the so-called reserve, antibiotics in settings like those and you'd breed resistant strains that no drugs could cure.

But all this was already happening, Jim said again and again. He talked about those patients in Peru who had come to Socios already resistant to second-line antibiotics, a couple of them with TB effectively resistant to every known anti-TB drug. The only way to prevent more of this was sound, well-financed MDR treatment, added on to DOTS. But while Jim believed in that argument, he knew he had to find a mechanism to ensure real control over cheaper drugs. He and Paul had just sent a young man to work at WHO in Geneva. Jim called him and explained the need for a control mechanism. "See if you can find a precedent," he said. A few days later the young man called to say he'd found one, an international entity called the Green Light Committee, established to control the distribution of meningococcal vaccine. "That's great!" said Jim. "Let's do the same thing. We'll create a committee to control second-line drugs."

"What do we call it?" asked the young PIH-er.

"Red Light Committee would be bad," said Jim. "How about Green Light Committee? That'll make it seem like we're just following precedent. "

The idea was simple. The committee would serve as the ultimate distributor for second-line drugs. Once prices fell, it would have real power. Any TB program that wanted low prices would have to prove to the committee that they had a good plan and a good underlying DOTS program, one that wouldn't breed further resistance. Most of "TB" endorsed the idea, and in a final compromise, WHO placed the second-line antibiotics in an annex to its essential drugs list.

The price reductions came in stages. By the year 2000, projects buying through the Green Light Committee paid about 95 percent less for four of the second-line drugs than they would have in 1996, and 84 percent less for two others. Howard Hiatt and Jim had persuaded Eli Lilly to donate large amounts of two antibiotics to PIH, and Lilly had promised to grant other MDR treatment projects vastly lowered prices. Capreomycin now cost ninety-eight cents a vial, 97 percent less than when Jim and Paul had first borrowed it from the pharmacy at the Brigham on their way to Peru. The drugs to treat a four-drug-resistant case of MDR now cost PIH about $1,500, instead of $15,000, and prices were still falling, substantially and rapidly. Arguments were far from over, but no one could say anymore that cost alone ruled out treating the disease in poor countries.

One member of WHO's TB division who had initially opposed the Green Light Committee took to describing himself as "the architect." Others had better claims to credit for the falling prices, including some members of Doctors Without Borders, to whom Jim and Paul had gone for help. But Guido Bakker, who was involved in most of the proceedings, told me, "I really see Jim as the one who really did this. He just pushed and pushed and pushed. Eighty-five percent of it was Jim."

═══

Since the start of the project in Lima, Jim and Paul had seen each other less and less frequently. They'd kept in touch mostly through e-mail.

But they met up at a TB meeting in Salzburg, Austria. Jim found it riveting, Paul nearly fell asleep. Afterward, they went out to dinner alone. Jim and Paul had always shared certain appetites. For telegraphic expression—"O for the P" instead of "a preferential option for the poor"—and action adventure movies and *People* magazine, which they called the Journal of Popular Studies, the JPS. They had similar diets, too. Dr. Farmer doused everything he ate with salt. Dr. Kim liked to say, "There are only two kinds of plants, stir-fryable and non." Not having had a chance to talk face-to-face in a while, they celebrated the occasion by ordering pizza.

Jim had a lot on his mind that evening. A few years back Paul had talked him into training as an infectious disease specialist. After a few months Jim had quit. He liked doctoring well enough, but Peru had introduced him to medicine on a different scale. It was the big issues surrounding health that excited him, he'd realized. He actually liked sitting for hours in conference rooms talking about operational research in international TB control. But he felt vaguely ashamed to admit that he wanted to have a hand in creating international health policy. As sometimes happened, Paul seemed to know what Jim was thinking.

"What do you want to do now?" he asked.

There was warmth in the question, Jim felt, a real invitation for him to come clean. "Political work is interesting to me, and it has to be done," he said. "I prefer it to taking care of patients. It's O for the P on an international scale."

"Well then, do it," Paul said.

"But didn't we always say that people who go into policy make a preferential option for their own ideas? For their own sorry asses?"

"Yeah, but, Jim, we trust you with power. We know you won't betray the poor."

Paul's self-assurance had sometimes seemed to fill all the space around him and Jim. In the old days, when Paul blew in from Haiti and wanted to talk to Jim but had to get to an appointment, he'd say, "Walk with me," as if everything on his agenda mattered more than anything Jim might have to do himself. For years Jim used to pick him up at the airport, but Paul never did that for him, not once. When they argued, which happened fairly often, Paul usually came out on top— or if he didn't, Jim often felt compelled to make him think he had. If Jim praised him, Paul was apt to say something like, "Thanks, Jimbo. I need to hear that." One time, when Jim replied, "Yeah, but why don't you ever say it to me?" Paul seemed surprised. "I do, don't I?"

Jim liked to say that he and Paul were "twin sons of different mothers." If so, Jim had been born second, and now, over pizza in Salzburg, he'd come of age, with Paul's blessing.

=

A lot of Farmer had rubbed off on Jim. Over the years their philosophical views had become virtually indistinguishable, especially on that set of notions which, it seemed to them, international health had adopted as scripture. Jim told me once, "There have been fundamental frame shifts in what human beings feel is morally defensible, what not. The world doesn't bind women's feet anymore, no one believes in slavery. Paul and I are anthropologists. We know that things change all the time. Culture changes all the time. Advertising people force changes in culture all the time. Why can't *we* do that? People in international health sit back and say, 'Will things change for the better? Who knows? But these Paul Farmers, they'll drop out, and when they do, we stalwarts will still be here figuring out the best way to spend two dollars and twenty-seven cents per capita for health care.' "

"Resources are always limited." In international health, this saying had great force. It lay behind most cost-effectiveness analyses. It often meant, "Be realistic." But it was usually uttered, Kim and Farmer felt, without any recognition of how, in a given place, resources had come to be limited, as if God had imposed poverty on places like Haiti. Strictly speaking, all resources everywhere were limited, Farmer would say in speeches. Then he'd add, "But they're less limited now than ever before in human history." That is, medicine now had the tools for stopping many plagues, and no one could say there wasn't enough money in the world to pay for them.

At PIH, though, the saying was true enough. They had spent several million of Tom White's dollars to buy the drugs for Peru. Ophelia had been hoarding up portions of the contributions PIH received, trying to create an endowment for the organization. She'd managed to put aside about a million dollars. Now it was gone, spent on Peru. And White was in his eighties and, as he'd planned, not very far from the end of his fortune. In early 2000 Ophelia, who was still in charge of the budget, wrote to Paul and Jim:

> Boys,
> We desperately need a big lump of cash. Basically, with 40k per month in salaries, 60k to Haiti, and 35k to Peru we can't make it on Tom's money. That is to say nothing of other expenses such as mortgage, health insurance, utilities blah blah blah. . . . Any ideas?

The three devised what they called "a disassembly strategy"—or, out of Tom White's earshot, "the post-Tom plan." Because of the falling prices of the second-line drugs, they could go on for a while treating patients in Lima, but in a year or two they'd have to stop. They'd also have to stop financing the research branch of PIH that Paul had founded years ago with his MacArthur money, and essentially remain a tiny private charity, struggling to support a health system in one corner of Haiti. "Screaming into the wilderness," as Jim put it.

Jim had an alternate vision, of course. In it, PIH would become an instrument for expanding the resources to treat TB, and in the process save itself. They had halted the spread of MDR in the shantytowns of northern Lima. Now they'd propose a project to wipe it out all over Peru. Then they'd go international. They'd show the world that it was possible to beat back that dread disease, and they'd show the world how to do it. And if MDR, then why not AIDS?

For over a year, Jim had been courting what he called "big-shot donors." None was bigger than the Gates Foundation. It had an endowment of roughly $22 billion, and it planned to spend about half the income, about $550 million a year, on projects to improve global health. Howard Hiatt had introduced Jim and Paul to the foundation's senior science adviser, a man named Bill Foege, one of the people responsible for the eradication of smallpox, known to favor unconventional approaches to supposedly impossible problems. Foege had encouraged them. So Jim started putting a grant proposal together. He met up with Paul again, this time in Moscow. They sat on the edges of their beds in a room at the Holiday Inn and talked about how much money to ask for. They argued a little. Paul thought two million dollars, maybe four.

"No," Jim said. "We're going to ask for forty-five million."

They'd never get that much, said Paul.

Borrowing one of Paul's favorite gambits in debate, Jim said, "On what data exactly do you base that statement?"

Part IV

A Light Month
for Travel

"Paul and Jim mobilized the world to accept drug-resistant TB as a soluble problem," Howard Hiatt told me one day in 2000, in his office at the Brigham. This was no small matter, he believed. "At least two million people a year die of TB. And when those people who die include large numbers of people with drug-resistant strains, as will happen unless a very big and good program gets established, it's not going to be two million. That number could be increased dramatically."

And MDR was only a part of an enormous problem in the world's health. TB and AIDS loomed over the new millennium. Add the malaria pandemic into the projections, and it seemed obvious that the world faced public health catastrophes on a scale not seen for centuries, since the eras of plague in Europe or the near extinctions of indigenous peoples in the Americas. Farmer, Hiatt seemed to say, should be solely engaged in the battle against those scourges, and at a level commensurate with their size. "The six months a year that Paul's looking after patients one-on-one in Haiti, if that time were converted to a major program for treating prisoners with TB in Russia and other eastern European countries, or malaria around the world, or AIDS in southern Africa—it doesn't matter where or what because you know he'll do important things. Because look at what he's done with only *part* of his time on MDR. Look what he's done with his skills and his political acumen! I have been urging him to take the role of consultant in Haiti and spend most of his time on worldwide projects."

Farmer was forty now, and he had the credentials to operate in the way Hiatt envisioned, on a purely executive level. In academic circles his reputation had grown. He was about to become a tenured Harvard professor. He was near the head of the line for the big prizes in medical anthropology; some of his peers were now saying that he'd "redefined" the field. As for his standing in clinical medicine, he'd become one of the doctors whom medical schools, in Europe as well as in the United States, invite to their campuses to deliver the lectures known as grand rounds. At the Brigham the surgeons had recently asked that he lecture to them, a signal honor not often granted to a mere medical doctor. He also sat on a number of councils in international health, and he'd made his views heard. But he didn't seem disposed to abandon any side of his work, including seeing patients one-on-one in Haiti.

It wasn't as though Farmer didn't want to do all he could to cure the world of poverty and disease. He just had his own ideas on how to go about it. Actually, he seemed to be the only person who understood the plan fully. A young assistant of his once said to him, in exasperation, that he had no priorities. That wasn't true, he replied. Patients came first, prisoners second, and students third. But you could see how the assistant might have felt lost in the details.

I liked to sit and watch him at his e-mail, in Cange and on airplanes and in airport waiting rooms. He had a way of moving a finger around in the air when he was thinking of how to make a point, and when he felt someone else had sniffed out a good one, he'd tap the side of his nose with an index finger. The e-mail itself was interesting to me. It conveyed some sense of his practice, a taste of its extent. In early 2000 he was receiving about seventy-five messages a day. He seemed to welcome most of them, and to have invited many. He answered the great majority.

There were consults on MDR patients in Peru, which he had to read and respond to carefully; worried and worrisome messages about projects in which PIH was involved, in Russia and Chiapas and Guatemala and Roxbury; affectionate greetings and requests for advice from priests and nuns and anthropologists and health bureaucrats and fellow doctors, in Cuba, London, Armenia, Sri Lanka, Paris, Indonesia, the Philippines, South Africa; and always a few queries like this: "Just a wrench to throw in your head. How would you like to work in Guinea-Bissau?" There were requests for counsel and for letters of recommendation, from youngsters who had worked as volunteers at PIH and now wanted to go to medical school, and from young doctors and epidemiologists who had in one way or another enlisted in the PIH cause. There were questions from his infectious disease fellow at the Brigham, and from a doctor in Boston who had been consulting him on the care of an indigent HIV patient, and from favorite medical students. "What is the mechanism/pathophys of acute hearing loss associated with meningitis?" one wrote.

Farmer answered promptly:

good morning, david. the damage from bacterial meningitis is ultimately due to the host inflammatory response. white cells. so that purulent meningitides that go for the base of the brain cause an almost mass-like inflammation there. now what courses under the base of the brain? the cranial nerves. and what do they do? permit little girls to hear. and what happens to them when they are surrounded with mass-like gelatinous inflammation (pus?) they get pinched. and they get anoxic. there goes hearing, and often ability to open both eyes, etc. even hydrocephalus is often due to inflammatory debris blocking the foramina. . . . it's anatomy, my friend. anatomy and pus. it's always anatomy and pus.

And when he was traveling, Creole e-mails flooded his account. I went with him once from Cange to the U.S. on a fund-raising trip of a day and a half. When we got back to Miami, en route to Haiti, and he checked his e-mail, this message was waiting for him, from one of the staff at Zanmi Lasante:

Dear Polo, we are so glad we will see you in a mere matter of hours. We miss you. We miss you as the dry, cracked earth misses the rain.

"After thirty-six hours?" Farmer said to his computer screen. "Haitians, man. They're totally over the top. My kind of people."

These days his life had one central logistical problem. Ophelia defined it succinctly: "Wherever he is, he's missing from somewhere." Farmer's solution for now was sleeping less and flying more. Early in 2000 I tagged along with him on what he called "a light month for travel."

We had spent two weeks in Cange, and in the midst of them had taken a quick trip to visit the church group in South Carolina. Now we were heading to Cuba for an AIDS conference. We'd spend the week after that in Moscow on TB business, with a stop in Paris en route.

"Who's paying your way?" I asked.

The church group, the Cuban government, and the Soros Foundation, he answered. He smiled. "Capitalists, commies, and Jesus Christers are paying."

⸻

When he was younger, Farmer used to come and go from Cange in jeans and a T-shirt, until he realized this upset his Haitian friends, who always dressed up to travel. Then Père Lafontant told him that if he was going off to represent them to the world, he should wear a suit. Farmer owned two but had loaned one to a friend. He preferred the black one anyway, because it allowed him, for example, to wipe the fuzz off the tip of his pen onto his pants leg while writing up orders at the Brigham, catch a night flight, say to Moscow or Lima, and still look presentable when he arrived.

We left Zanmi Lasante for the airport around dawn. Ten Cangeois climbed on board, cramming themselves into the cab of the truck and among the suitcases in the open bed in the rear. Farmer, dressed in his suit, issued a bunch of last-minute requests and instructions to the staff who came to see him off, and got into the driver's seat—he suffered from motion sickness, and being at the wheel lessened his nausea—and the truck, like a small boat leaving its harbor, departed the smooth pavement of the complex and began lurching down National Highway 3.

It was early. We hadn't eaten breakfast. My back felt wrenched already. I was narrating Haiti on my own, in my mind, bouncing up and down in the cab of the truck. This so-called road had been built early in the twentieth century, during the first American occupation of Haiti. The U.S. Marines had supervised its construction. To get the job done, they'd revived an institution known as the *corvée,* a system of conscript labor that dated back to slavery days. The peasants of the central plateau staged an insurrection, which the Marines put down violently. In a book Farmer had shown me, there was a photograph of a conscripted and presumably recalcitrant roadworker who had been disciplined by the Marine-supervised Haitian *gendarmes.* In the photograph, the man lies on the ground with both hands cut off.

Sights along this roadside were less dramatic now but brutal enough for 6:00 A.M.—the emaciated beggars, the barefoot children lugging water. Through the jouncing windshield, I saw a thin man in a straw hat on a starving Haitian pony. He was mounted on a traditional Haitian saddle, made of straw, designed, it would seem, to abrade the backs of donkeys and ponies until they bled. He was kicking the pony's protruding ribs, hurrying, I imagined, to get to work on some rocky, infertile piece of local farmland so his children could have at least one meal today. I was looking around in my mind for a consoling way to view the roadside sights and also, frankly, for something likely to impress Farmer. A fragment from my religious education bubbled up. I said, "If you've done it unto the least of them, you've done it unto me."

"Matthew twenty-five," said Farmer. "Inasmuch as you have done it unto the least of these my brethren, you have done it unto me." He went on, paraphrasing, "When I was hungry, you fed me. When I was thirsty, you gave me something to drink. When I was a stranger, you took me in. When I was naked, you gave me clothes. When I was sick, when I was in prison, you visited me. *Then* it says, Inasmuch as you did it *not,* you're screwed." He smiled, swerving around another giant rut in the road.

The conversation was desultory, and the ride uneventful, until we came to the descent of Morne Kabrit, the view opening below us of the once fertile and now alkalized Cul-de-Sac Plain and beyond it Port-au-Prince. This was the most dangerous part of the road, *kwazman* territory. Farmer defined the term for me: "When you encounter another truck or something like that boulder we just glanced off and it ain't good, that's a *kwazman*." The aftermath of a *kwazman* lay up ahead, a truck turned onto its side along the inner edge of the road, not far from the spot where Paul and Ophelia had come upon the dead mango lady seventeen years before. Farmer stopped and peered at the wreck through the windshield. But there were no people around the wreck, no bodies on the ground this time. "It doesn't look like anyone got hurt," he said in English to me, then in Creole to the Cangeois in the back.

One of the men replied, "Well, someone in that truck could have had a general curse on him, and he might have taken the occasion to die."

Farmer translated this for me and laughed and, still laughing, drove on. His first stop was the jail in Croix des Bouquets, a Port-au-Prince suburb. An unchecked *bwat* on his current list of things to do read, "Prison extraction." One of the men in the back of the truck, a peasant farmer from Kay Epin, had a son who had left home to work as a security guard in the city; recently, the young man had been jailed on suspicion of murder. Farmer had already arranged for a lawyer. He was stopping at the jail so that the father could speak to his son.

The sergeant at the desk said, "You're not allowed in." Farmer put a hand on the sergeant's shoulder and talked his way past. The cell where the young man languished was unlit. In the shadows within you could see a crowd of at least thirty young men. Nearer the light, a dozen faces peered out through the bars. "Hi," said Farmer.

"Hi, Doc," many voices replied. Several raised their hands and wiggled their fingers. A fierce odor came out—dried sweat, foul breath, urine, and shit. The son stood at the bars and talked to his father. Then the father stood back and gazed at his boy. Farmer spoke to the young man for a while, telling him about the lawyer.

We went outside. The truck wouldn't start. The passengers from Cange and I climbed out and pushed. The engine caught. We climbed back in. "So much for the white knight making his departure," said Farmer. "When I was sick, when I was in prison, when I needed clothes, you gave me, et cetera. We got those covered." He went on, "One thing that comes back to me, with all this cost-efficacy crap, if I saved one patient in my whole life, that wouldn't be too bad. What did you do with your life? I saved Michela, got a guy out of jail. So I'm lucky." He added, "To have a chance to save a zillion of them, I dig that."

After an errand downtown, he drove to the airport. The closer we got, the thicker the crowds of women and children hawking sodas and fruit and geegaws among the rubble by the side of the road. Up ahead Farmer spotted a broken-down car, the occupants outside and pushing. He drove around it. "Am I sinning? But Matthew twenty-five doesn't say anything about . . ." He lifted his voice and sang: "When my car broke down, you gave me a push." The traffic was snarled as usual. Crowds always thronged the airport when a big plane was coming or going, and most of the people seemed to have no business there except hope. It wasn't just taxi drivers looking for fares who gathered at this seam in the world but children and old men and women leaning on sticks and people with missing limbs, all straining at the barricades, shouting and waving at the arriving passengers. On a wall of the main terminal Farmer spotted a sign in English, placed there for tourists during the last holiday season:

BEST WISHES FOR THE CHRISTMAS
AND HAPPINESS FOR THE NEW MILLENNIUM 2000

Beneath this was a painting of a reindeer. "Oh," said Farmer. "An example of the local fauna. The poor Haitians. God bless the Haitians. They try so hard."

═══

My gloom lifted on the airplane, but Farmer, I was learning, found it hard to leave Haiti. "You and I, we can leave whenever we want. But most Haitians are never going to get to go anywhere, you know?" he'd said as we boarded. A little later, when the plane banked over the Bay of Port-au-Prince, he glanced out the window once, then turned his face away. For a minute or two the central plateau was laid out in the window beside him, a brown landscape dotted with just a little green, eroded mountainsides that looked like the ribs of starving animals, and rivers that stained the turquoise waters brown, bleeding the last of Haiti's topsoil into the sea. "It bothers me even to look at it," Farmer said, narrating Haiti for what would be the last time in a while. "It can't support eight million people, and there they are. There they are, kidnapped from West Africa."

He went to work on thank-you notes to PIH contributors. Finishing five, he got to check off a *bwat*. This cheered him up. But then lunch was served, and I was about to start eating when I looked over and saw that his fold-down tray was empty. "Hey, where's your meal?"

"Maybe they know about the kid," said Farmer. "That I failed to save her."

A little girl had died in the Children's Pavilion last night, one he felt shouldn't have. This was the first I'd heard of it. He'd stayed up all night, trying every trick he knew to save her.

"I'm sorry," I said.

"There's a lot of death in Haiti," he answered. "Sometimes I get so fucking sick of it, babies dying . . ." His lunch had arrived by now. He ate some of it, then said, "Let's go over the patients." He went bed by bed through the TB hospital, the main hospital, the Children's Pavilion. "And there's the preemie who worried me because she's no bigger than a peanut. But she looked fine." He was smiling, finally. "For a tadpole."

When we landed in Miami, Farmer surveyed the cabin. He figured about 20 percent of our fellow passengers had never flown before. He could point them out—the very thin ones, the ones with callused hands and faces, the men who looked self-consciously dressed up, as if for the first time, the women in dresses that were covered with ruffles. "We're about to see something horrible."

"What?"

"The escalators."

He stood near the top of the first. A while ago he had gone to the airport administration to ask them to do something about the problem, but evidently they hadn't listened. Every fourth or fifth Haitian would come to a stop at the head of the escalator and look down at the moving stairs. They'd pause as if at the edge of deep water, and then start to run, trying to match the speed of their legs with the apparent speed of the stairs. "Don't run. Hold on to the rail," Farmer called in Creole to an elderly-looking woman about to tip over. She regained her balance. He turned to me, his face grim again. "The more ruffles, the more stumbles."

===

Ophelia thought that Paul had a fairly complex personality, built of oppositions—a need for frenzied activity that verged, she thought, on desperation, and a towering self-confidence oddly combined with a hunger for affirmation. He was always asking, "How am I doin'?" and if she didn't praise him, he'd be hurt. She thought she understood; he took on more than he could fix, so of course he wanted reassurance. And yet he also seemed "terribly simple." She thought he had never experienced true depression, a freedom so enviable she almost resented it. "I've never known despair and I don't think I ever will," he wrote me once. It was as if in seeking out suffering in some of the world's most desperate locales, he made himself immune to the self-consuming varieties of psychic pain. He'd told me back in Haiti, "I may be a more sunny, cheerful person than you. No one believes that I'm cheerful because of what I say and write, but I only say and write those things because they're true." He was often sad, of course, but it didn't take much to cheer him up.

Miami Airport was his usual hub. Many business travelers rated it one of their least favorite. Not Farmer. Depending on its length, a layover there was either "a Miami day" or "a Miami day plus," and both included a haircut from his favorite Cuban barber—they'd chat in Spanish—and the purchase of the latest issue of *People* magazine, the JPS. And then it was up to the Admirals' Club, which he was in the habit of calling "Amirales." There he'd take a hot shower, then stake out a section of lounge—this was "making a cave" or "getting cavea-ceous at Amirales"—and answer e-mail from a soft easy chair while sipping a glass of red wine. Today was a Miami day plus, which meant that, in addition to all those other exquisite pleasures, we stayed the night in the airport hotel.

Farmer spent an hour that evening locating the gate for our charter flight to Havana. He had a brand-new young assistant back in Boston, but it seemed that the assistant had joined Partners In Health to do so-cial justice work, not to be a travel agent. This was a common sort of problem in the organization, as in any that relies heavily on volunteers and can't pay its salaried employees much. When it came to managing personnel, Ophelia and Jim had at least one other special handicap. No one could be fired—Farmer's rule—except for stealing or slap-ping a patient twice. The rule used to be one slap and you were out, but then an employee in Cange hit a patient, and rather than fire the guilty party, Farmer amended the rule. "Two slaps," he insisted.

His young assistant deserved some sympathy. These days a seem-ingly endless line of people wanted some of Farmer's time, and he didn't like to turn anyone down. Farmer had a habit of complaining that he had no time off and then, when some was scheduled, of filling it with a meeting or a speaking engagement. No one had ever been able to order his affairs flawlessly. His last assistant, a woman in her thirties, had come close. But he had promoted her.

That night in the hotel, Farmer got up to go to the bathroom and, not wanting to wake me, left the lights off. He smashed his toe into a suitcase in the dark. When we got up at 4:00 A.M., the toe had turned purple. He diagnosed a fracture but limped along through the termi-nal without complaint, his computer bag over a shoulder, his latest wallet—a plastic shopping bag—in one hand and in the other his suit-case. It contained just a smattering of clothes—only three shirts for two weeks—but was jammed full with slides for lectures and with presents for his Cuban hosts. "Do you think I like wearing the same shirt five days in a row?" he once asked me. I thought that at times he probably did. At times he'd seem to say that if the world weren't in such terrible shape and its leaders would only do their jobs, he wouldn't have to suffer such discomforts. But complaint didn't seem to be his usual mode. He said the choice between, for instance, carrying extra shirts and carrying medicines was easy. "The trick is," he said, "to keep your body clean and change your underwear." I would learn that he had many such tricks. "Traveler's tip number one thousand seventy-three. If you don't have time to eat, and there's no other food on the plane, a package of peanuts and Bloody Mary mix are six hundred calories." This morning I carried the presents that didn't fit in his bag. He was very grateful. I think he felt obliged to keep getting presents until he had more than he could easily carry. Then he'd know he had enough.

I remarked on his sleepless nights, his hundred-hour weeks, his incessant travel, as he hobbled along.

He said, "The problem is, if I don't work this hard, someone will die who doesn't have to. That sounds megalomaniacal. I wouldn't have said that to you before I'd taken you to Haiti and you had seen that it was manifestly true." He added earnestly, "But I do want to get into better shape. I did my push-ups this morning." He had, in fact, done a set of upward-facing push-ups between two chairs, so as to protect his toe.

Up ahead we could see the check-in point for the charter flight to Havana. You could tell from the piles of luggage, the boxes containing radios and kitchen appliances, the sacks full of things like disposable diapers. The scene resembled the ones at ticket counters serving flights to Haiti, except that the piles here weren't as mountainous or the suitcases as dilapidated. One can guess a lot about the economic condition of a country by inspecting the baggage people carry there from the United States, the shopping mall for the poor countries of the world. This sort of scene, I think, was so commonplace to Farmer as not to be worth remarking on. For going on eighteen years he'd been performing for Haitians what are called *commission*, Creole for "I got some stuff for you to carry on the plane." "They're the story of Paul's life," Jim Kim told me. " 'I have an uncle who lives in Poughkeepsie, can you bring this mango to him?' Or 'Can you buy me a watch in the

States? Can you buy me a radio and take this piece of bread to my aunt in Brooklyn?' And Paul will say, 'Sure.' "

After we checked in, we sat at an airport restaurant table, and Farmer worked on more thank-you notes. He was smiling, and I figured he was looking forward to Cuba, because he said, "No dead babies for a while."

CHAPTER 21

When the plane descended toward Havana, Farmer stared intently out the window, making exclamations. "Look! Only ninety miles from Haiti and look! Trees! Crops! It's all so verdant. At the height of the dry season! The same ecology as Haiti's, and look!"

The Cuban doctor who was running the AIDS conference, an old friend of Farmer's named Jorge Pérez, had sent a car for him. On the ride into Havana, I got my first glimpse of a Cuban political billboard, a gigantically enlarged version of the famous photograph of Che Guevara in a beret, and I was reminded that an American who found anything good to say about Cuba under Castro still ran the risk of being labeled a communist stooge. I knew Farmer was fond of Cuba, not mainly, I thought, for ideological reasons but because of its health statistics—statistics vetted by WHO and generally regarded as among the most accurate in the world.

Many things affect a public's health, of course—nutrition and transportation, crime and housing, pest control and sanitation, as well as medicine. In Cuba, life expectancies were about the same as in the United States. Since its revolution Cuba had achieved real control over diseases still burgeoning ninety miles away in Haiti, such as dengue fever, typhoid, tuberculosis, AIDS. Later, accompanying Dr. Pérez on rounds at his hospital, the national infectious disease hospital, we would come to the room of a patient with malaria, and Pérez would announce that his young doctors had missed the initial diagnosis because they'd never seen a case of malaria before. And here was

Farmer, who had stood, time after time for eighteen years, at the bed-sides of Haitian peasants just arrived by donkey in the last throes of cerebral malaria—grandparents, mothers, fathers, children—already in convulsions.

"For me to admire Cuban medicine is a given," Farmer said. It was a poor country, and made that way at least in part by the United States' long embargo, yet when the Soviet Union had dissolved and Cuba had lost both its patron and most of its foreign trade, the regime had listened to the warnings of its epidemiologists and had actually in-creased expenditures on public health. By American standards Cuban doctors lacked equipment, and even by Cuban standards they were poorly paid, but they were generally well-trained, and Cuba had more of them per capita than any other country in the world—more than twice as many as the United States. Everyone, it appeared, had access to their services, and to procedures like open heart surgery. Indeed, ac-cording to a study by WHO, Cuba had the world's most equitably dis-tributed medicine. Moreover, Cuba seemed to have mostly abandoned its campaign to change the world by exporting troops. Now they were sending doctors instead, to dozens of poor countries. About five hun-dred Cuban doctors worked gratis in Haiti now—not very effectively, because they lacked equipment, but even as a gesture it meant a lot to Farmer.

One time he got in an argument about Cuba with some friends of his, fellow Harvard professors, who said that the Scandinavian coun-tries offered the best examples of how to provide both excellent pub-lic health and political freedom. Farmer said they were talking about managing wealth. He was talking about managing poverty. Haiti was a bad example of how to do that. Cuba was a good one.

He had studied the world's ideologies. The Marxist analysis, which liberation theology borrowed, seemed to him undeniably accurate. How could anyone say that no war among socioeconomic classes ex-isted, or that suffering wasn't a "social creation," especially now, when humanity had developed a grand array of tools to alleviate suffering. And he was more interested in denouncing the faults of the capitalist world than in cataloging the failures of socialism. "We should all be criticizing the excesses of the powerful, if we can demonstrate so readily that these excesses hurt the poor and vulnerable." But years ago he'd concluded that Marxism wouldn't answer the questions posed by the suffering he encountered in Haiti. And he had quarrels with the Marxists he'd read: "What I don't like about Marxist litera- ture is what I don't like about academic pursuits—and isn't that what Marxism is, now? In general, the arrogance, the petty infighting, the dishonesty, the desire for self-promotion, the orthodoxy. I can't stand the orthodoxy, and I'll bet that's one reason that science did not flour- ish in the former Soviet Union."

He distrusted all ideologies, including his own, at least a little. "It's an ology, after all," he had written to me about liberation theology. "And all ologies fail us at some point. At a point, I suspect, not very far from where the Haitian poor live out their dangerous lives." Where might it fail? He told me, "If one pushes this ology to its logical con- clusion, then God is to be found in the struggle against injustice. But if the odds are so preposterously stacked against the poor—machetes versus Uzis, donkeys versus tanks, stones versus missiles, or even ty- phoid versus cancer—then is it responsible, is it wise, to push the poor to claim what is theirs by right? What happens when the destitute in Guatemala, El Salvador, Haiti, wherever, are moved by a rereading of the Gospels to stand up for what is theirs, to reclaim what was theirs and was taken away, to ask only that they enjoy decent poverty rather than the misery we see here every day in Haiti? We know the answer to that question, because we are digging up their bodies in Guatemala."

For me, the first sights of communist Cuba were a great relief after Haiti. Paved roads and old American cars, instead of litters on the *gwo wout la*. Cuba had food rationing and allotments of coffee adulterated with ground peas, but no starvation, no enforced malnutrition. I no- ticed a group of prostitutes on one main road, and housing projects in need of paint and repair, like most buildings in Havana. But I still had in mind the slums of Port-au-Prince and the huts of the central plateau, and Cuba looked lovely to me.

When we got to our hotel, Farmer said, "I can sleep here. Everyone here has a doctor." He lay down on his bed and within a few minutes he was asleep.

===

"I relish the break from Haiti," Farmer told me when he woke up. "I mean, I feel guilty. I feel guilty leaving, but I'm going to try to raise money for Haiti while I'm here." He was counting on Dr. Pérez for some help.

Pérez was in his mid-fifties. The top of his head reached roughly the altitude of Farmer's bony shoulders. Farmer said that when he first laid eyes on Pérez, some years before, a very tall patient was wagging a finger in Jorge's face, saying in Spanish, "Listen to me, you. I have a problem with you." And Pérez was looking up at the man and nodding. Farmer said he remembered thinking, "That looks like a good doctor-patient relationship." They'd been friends ever since.

Farmer was looking in Cuba, first of all, for money to stockpile antiretroviral drugs, enough to treat twenty-five patients with full-blown AIDS back in Cange—twenty-five patients for starters. At the AIDS conference he met a woman who might be able to help, if she would. She was in charge of the United Nations' project on HIV/AIDS, UNAIDS, for the Caribbean. He lobbied her over several days. He gave her a copy of *Infections and Inequalities,* and inscribed it, "For Peggy McAvoy with a big hug of solidarity and with high hopes for your help in Haiti." He said to me, "My subtlety. No one gives guilt trips like I give." At the cocktail party, full of all sorts of medical dignitaries, he tried to close the sale, and it seemed as though he had, with a little help from Dr. Pérez, who approached and told Peggy, speaking of Farmer, "He is a friend of mine." She asked Farmer for a written proposal. And Farmer said, his face bright, "Can I give you a kiss? Can I give you two?"

He also hoped to begin to solve one of Zanmi Lasante's most persistent problems. All but one of the Haitian doctors who worked in Cange had their homes in Port-au-Prince, or abroad—in Canada or Florida or New Jersey. They were "middle-class Haitians," Farmer explained. "And middle-class Haitians regard Cange as an uninhabitable place, *nan raje,* in the sticks." To work out in the central plateau away from their families, where there was nothing to do but work and play Ping-Pong—Farmer had recently bought the doctors a Ping-Pong table—had proved too great a sacrifice for many over the years. Several, most recently his gynecologist, had gone to work in the States, and some of those had clearly gone to work for Farmer with that aim in mind, to be trained by Doktè Paul, then to emigrate, and he always felt obliged to help them leave. So he hoped to begin creating some doctors indigenous to Cange. He and his Haiti staff had picked out two local youths. Farmer hoped to send them to the huge new medical school that Cuba was opening for Latin American students.

He told Dr. Pérez about this plan, and Pérez arranged a private meeting between Farmer and the secretary of Cuba's Council of State, a medical doctor named José Miyar Barruecos, known as Choumy. A distinguished-looking man, in his sixties I figured.

They talked for a while, and then in Spanish Farmer asked, "Can I send you two students this year?"

"From the U.S.?"

"No, Haiti."

"Por supuesto," said Choumy. "Of course."

Luc Montagnier, the man generally credited with discovering the human immunodeficiency virus, was speaking at the conference. This meant of course that the French ambassador to Cuba would show up at some point. When he did, Farmer got his ear and also Montagnier's. Looking on, I thought they seemed surprised, then impressed by Farmer's French. He told them he dreamed of a new kind of "triangle," doctors from Cuba and money from France coming together in Haiti. He was of course playing on the term *triangular trade,* the trade that had created the French slave colony that had turned into Haiti. He invited Montagnier to Cange, and after some hesitation Montagnier said he would come. The ambassador told Farmer, "Yes, we too are going to help with the Haitians."

Polite and worthless promises maybe, but Farmer in the role of supplicant seemed artfully ingenuous. Assume that each new promise was real and obtain as many as possible, to increase the odds that one or two might be real. And he'd follow up with calls, letters, e-mails, and if those didn't bring results, they still might produce a little shame, which might increase the chances that the next promise would be real.

Farmer also had formal duties in Cuba. He was scheduled to give two talks at the conference. "What are the subjects?" I asked.

"One speech is for clinicians, how to deal with HIV and TB coinfection," he said. "The other is why life sucks."

He began the second speech by saying, "Today I'm going to talk about the problem of a more important coinfection, which is poverty. Poverty and inequality." Up on the screen in the ampitheater of Cuba's infectious disease hospital, beside the tall, reedy fellow in the black suit, the blue waters of the Péligre Reservoir appeared. "Now, in this country where I have worked for eighteen years, the *campesinos* lost their land to a hydroelectric dam."

=

Farmer asked the audience to remember the days when expert opinion had retailed all sorts of nonsense about who caught HIV and why, the days when to be Haitian was to be part of a "risk group." He and his staff had designed a study in Cange, he said, to try to get at the local facts. Two hundred women were involved, half infected with HIV, half not. Almost none in either group had been exposed to risks often mentioned in expert commentary—intramuscular injections, blood transfusions, intravenous drug use. Around Cange, Farmer noted, the peasants' vocabulary didn't even contain a word for illicit drugs, which virtually no one there could afford anyway. And none of the women had been especially promiscuous; on average, they'd had sexual relations with two different men, consecutively not concurrently, practicing "serial monogamy." Between the groups of women, only two differences stood out. Unlike the uninfected, many of the ones with AIDS had worked as servants in Port-au-Prince. Obviously, domestic service hadn't given them HIV, but it did describe their economic desperation—working for Haiti's elite was rarely pleasant or remunerative. Uniformly, the infected women named that kind of desperation, deep poverty and illiteracy, as their reason for having taken what appeared to be the real risk for AIDS, which was cohabiting with truck drivers or soldiers.

"Why those two groups of men?" Farmer asked from the podium. Were they known to be sexier than other Haitian men? Of course not. What they had were steady jobs, in an economy where an official unemployment rate of 70 percent probably understated the case. Truck drivers were mobile and could keep women in many ports. And soldiers, back in those days of military rule, had wielded a special coercive power over every peasant.

Up at the podium, Farmer went on with the story: After the study was done, he returned to the United States and logged on to MEDLINE. He entered "AIDS," and the names of thousands of studies came up on his computer screen. Then he entered "AIDS and women," and only a handful of studies appeared. "And when I crossed 'AIDS, women, and poverty,' the message said, 'There are no studies meeting those specifications.' "

Farmer extended a hand toward the screen behind him, now filled with a gigantically enlarged graph of the study from Cange. "There are reasons why people are uncomfortable talking about this. Fine. But if we want to stop AIDS, we better find out about this. Countries with the steepest grades of inequality and the greatest poverty have the biggest AIDS problems, and I'm sure Professor Montagnier would agree that while coinfections are important cofactors, they're not as important as these. We need to erase social inequalities, and very few countries have done that." He closed in one of his favorite ways, by quoting a peasant. "A woman in Cange said to me, 'You want to stop HIV in women? Give them jobs.' "

By now I felt I was getting a sense of how Farmer put together experience and philosophy. In trying to control TB and AIDS in the central plateau, he had ended up wrangling, not much with third world myths, like beliefs in sorcery, but usually with first world ones, like expert theories that exaggerated the power poor women had to protect themselves from AIDS. This was Cuba, of course, the hemisphere's small, lonely iconoclast. The amphitheater, about half full, gave him a long, loud round of applause.

————

Farmer told me he'd like to hang out at the conference, but he spent less time there than in our hotel room, lying on his bed, a pillow behind his head, a pillow under his knees, his computer on his lap. Once in a while he'd begin to doze, then jump up and pace the floor, swinging his arms, saying to himself, "Come on, Pel. Come on." He typed away. At the proposal for UNAIDS, at a different grant proposal for obtaining antiretroviral medicines for Zanmi Lasante (you could never seek out too many sources of funding when you didn't have funding), at a countereditorial he'd been asked to write in response to an editorial questioning the wisdom of treating MDR-TB in Russia. "Who's it for?" I asked.

"*The Journal of Tuberculosis and Lung Disease,*" he said, typing away. "I'm sure you get it at home."

From time to time he worked on his new book, *Pathologies of Power.* He had a bound typescript of the rough draft. It contained a chapter comparing the two ways in which AIDS had been managed on the island of Cuba—the Cuban approach and the American quarantine of HIV-positive Haitian refugees, conducted in the early nineties on the Guantánamo naval base. In the room Farmer read aloud from a book by a respected American political scientist who had also compared the two quarantines, calling them roughly equivalent. "It makes my blood boil," said Farmer.

He didn't approve of quarantine for AIDS. "Quarantine has never been shown to be an effective measure in controlling sexually transmitted diseases," he said. He went on, "Both Guantánamo and Cuba's AIDS sanitorium were quarantines. But it's a *lie* to say they weren't different."

He had interviewed some of the Haitians quarantined on Guantánamo, and from them heard stories of wretched treatment at the hands of the U.S. military—of food with maggots in it, of compulsory blood tests and compulsory injections of the long-acting contraceptive Depo-Provera—its effects can last up to eighteen months—of beatings when they protested. One didn't have to take the Haitians' word for all of this. In 1993 an American federal judge had described the quarantine in harsh terms and ended it, ruling it unconstitutional.

The other quarantine of HIV patients in Cuba, the Cuban government's, had been conducted in a place called Santiago de las Vegas. It lay about an hour's drive from Havana. Dr. Pérez had played a big part in its history. He took us there in his battered Russian Lada sedan.

I enjoyed looking out at the countryside, all colored for me by contrast with Haiti's—the electric power wires, the irrigated fields. We turned off the highway onto a narrower paved road, and after a while Dr. Pérez announced, "We are arriving now to the concentration camp. You will see the concentration camp we have here." That was what the AIDS sanatorium had been called in a *New York Times* op-ed.

On the right lay the grounds of what had clearly been a grand estate. We turned down the drive. A bare-chested, heavily muscled young man wearing a black beret was coming out the gate on a bicycle. "Please stop," said Farmer to Pérez's driver. Then Farmer jumped out and called to the bicyclist, "Eduardo!" And Eduardo did a double take, climbed off his bike, grinning, then enveloped Farmer in a hug. He was a former Cuban soldier who had contracted AIDS in Africa, a patient of Pérez's. Farmer had met Eduardo on a previous trip and had doctored him a little. I never heard Farmer complain of having too many patients, and it seemed clear that he couldn't feel comfortable anywhere not having any at all. So in Cuba he borrowed some from Pérez.

Farmer climbed back in, and we drove on, up to an old hacienda. A wealthy Cuban had owned it, and fled during the revolution. The interior was high-ceilinged, many-roomed. Stains darkened the walls here and there, but the place wasn't exactly shabby. It had the feeling of a defrocked place, where you'd find a gray filing cabinet in a spot designed for a mahogany highboy.

During lunch in the headquarters building, Dr. Pérez told us his version of the history of the sanatorium. He said that he and his boss, Gustavo Kouri, were giving Fidel Castro a report about malaria in

Africa when Castro asked, "What are you going to do to stop AIDS from entering Cuba?"

Pérez went on: "Gustavo said, 'AIDS has no importance.' Then Fidel tugged his beard and said, 'You don't know what you're talking about. It's going to be the disease of the century, and it is your responsibility, Gustavo, to stop AIDS from spreading in Cuba.' "

The Cuban authorities had decided to quarantine people infected with HIV at this old hacienda, under military discipline—first soldiers and then a combustible mixture of soldiers and homosexual men, nastiest no doubt for the gay inmates, although everyone was well-fed and got medical treatment. When Pérez took over a few years later, he let in visitors, had the tall surrounding wall torn down—"Because reporters came here and they were climbing trees"—and little by little changed the rules, first allowing patients to leave on passes once they'd shown they could be trusted to practice safe sex, and eventually lifting the quarantine altogether. Pérez said he'd imagined that all the patients would leave at that point, but only 20 percent did, in part because conditions at the sanatorium were generally better than elsewhere.

Dr. Pérez led us on a tour of the patients' quarters, little houses and apartments set among gardens and palm trees. The settlement looked like a working-class American suburb. We visited the patient Eduardo's house—three little rooms. On the bureau stood a snapshot of Farmer. Paul spotted it and stared, his face turning red. When he recovered, he said to Eduardo, "I see you're still smoking cigarettes." Eduardo offered him the pack, and Farmer pushed it aside, laughing. "No. I was about to say you should quit."

The tour resumed. Farmer kept remarking on how pleasant and peaceful these quarters were, and finally I said to him, "I find them kind of depressing."

"Really?" He seemed surprised. "Compared to what I grew up in, it's pretty nice. They have gas stoves, air-conditioning, electricity, TV." Actually, it wasn't the sanatorium's housing that troubled me. I felt that Farmer was suspending his usually sharp critical judgment. I thought he was looking only for things to praise. So I was doing the opposite. Maybe I just wanted an argument. He didn't, clearly. He let the subject drop.

As we walked around, I told myself it was too easy to pass judgment now on the way various societies had responded to AIDS in the first panicky years of a terrifying public health emergency. And it was probably facile to compare the responses of the United States and Cuba. The countries were so different in size and complexity. But I had to wonder if I would have felt the same reserve if the outcomes had been reversed. By 2000 the overall rates of HIV infection and deaths from AIDS were dropping in the United States, but infections and deaths had claimed a much larger percentage of the population than in Cuba, and HIV had become mainly a heterosexual disease concentrated among the American poor. Cuba, meanwhile, had the lowest per capita incidence of HIV in the Western Hemisphere—its HIV statistics were probably among the most accurate in the world, for the simple reason that, in Cuba, testing wasn't optional and millions had been tested. On an island of 11 million, only 2,669 had tested positive as of 2000. The virus had progressed to AIDS in 1,003 of those people, and 653 had died. Only five children had caught HIV from their mothers, and all those children were still alive. Because Cuba had acted quickly to clean up its blood supply, only 10 people had contracted HIV from transfusions. One could argue that the U.S. embargo had protected the island, but then again, back at the start of the epidemic Cuba had engaged in a lot of commerce with Africa.

We drove back toward Havana. Pérez said he'd gotten a call that morning from the Barbados embassy. They wanted him to see the daughter of the ambassador. "But I don't know even who she is. They phoned me five times yesterday. Anyway, I am with Paul Farmer today."

Farmer and Pérez seemed to share one favorite recreation, which was visiting patients. When Pérez came to Boston, he liked to go on rounds with Farmer. Not long after we'd arrived in Havana, Farmer had asked, "Are we going to see some patients, Jorge?"

"Well, of course."

Pérez also took him to meet Cuba's chief forensic pathologist, the person who had led the team that had found Che Guevara's secret grave in Bolivia—or claimed to have found it, some would say. The pathologist stood up at his desk to tell the story, in a loud voice, at moments practically declaiming, recounting how they had done mathematical modeling, employed their own Cuban archaeologist, soil chemist, geologist, and botanist, and how, after searching for three hundred days, they had finally come upon the bones and identified them and sneaked them back to Cuba. "We were finding heroes. I was finding *my* heroes. As a researcher, as a scientist, and because of the revolution, we were proud. It is very important for the revolution. It is a mixture. That and doing your job."

We went to dinner at Pérez's house, which was about as large and well-furnished as a unit in a decent American housing development—Farmer made sure I noticed that Pérez's driver ate with the family. Another night we had dinner in a restaurant said to have been one of Hemingway's favorites—there were probably almost as many of those in Havana as in Key West—men with guitars surrounding the table to sing "El Comandante," the mournful ballad of Che. At the hotel Farmer got to do variations of hortitorture. There were some cockatoos in a cage in the lobby. Going in and coming out, he always stopped to gaze at them. "They're Psittaciformes, by the way. I know that because they're associated with a disease called psittacosis." The hotel also had a fish tank and several small fish ponds, over which he'd bend his lanky torso, naming species. "Blue gourami, black molly, neon tetra, orange barb."

Cuba really was a holiday, by his standards. In almost every other place where he worked, in Siberia, in the central plateau of Haiti, in the northern slums of Lima, in Chiapas under siege, he could send and receive e-mail. But in Cuba, because of the embargo, he was cut off from his usual electronic routine. He'd pay for this later, but for the moment he was relieved of the requests and duties that e-mail brought him every day, anywhere else but in Cuba.

He had traveled more than anyone I knew, and seen fewer of the brochure sights. He'd never been to Machu Picchu in Peru. He'd never gone to the Bolshoi in Moscow. He didn't go sightseeing in Cuba either. On this trip, most of what he saw of old Havana he glimpsed through the windows of Dr. Pérez's Lada. A city like a tarnished heirloom, pleasing—from the outside looking in, at least—in the half decay of its sculpted cornices, arcades, and porticoes, and loveliest in the warm, windy evenings, when the waves crashed against the seawall, raining spray on lovers along the Malecón. But it was as if Farmer had built himself an alarm system by which every pleasant thing set off a recording saying, "You're forgetting Haiti." He stared out at the monumental banyan trees along a route that Pérez's driver took, and said softly, "I've worked eighteen years in Haiti, and everything has gotten worse."

"We haven't done enough yet in Haiti," he told me at one point.

"What about Zanmi Lasante?"

"Zanmi Lasante *is* an oasis, the best thing of its kind in Haiti. But it's not as good as here. The Cubans would have done a better job."

=

Again and again during our stop in Cuba, Farmer had marveled at the attentions lavished on him. Dr. Pérez had a hospital and a conference to run, and he had to entertain a surefire Nobel Prize–winner-to-be in Luc Montagnier. And yet he'd spent a large part of every day and all his evenings with Farmer. One night in the hotel room, Farmer looked up from his computer and asked me what I thought accounted for this.

It seemed to me that he rarely asked a question for which he didn't have the answer. So, to keep the peace, I should have tried to find the one he had in mind. Instead, I told Farmer I imagined that the Cubans liked his published attacks on American policy in Latin America, his frank admiration of Cuban public health and medicine, his efforts to create connections between Harvard and Cuba. I added, "And Jorge constantly introduces you by saying, 'He is my friend.' "

I looked over and found Farmer's pale blue eyes fixed on me. The Farmer stare. It could make you think he was examining an X ray of your soul or, if you were irritated with him, that he imagined he was examining one. My eyes wanted to look away, and I wasn't going to let them.

"I get the same reception everywhere," he said. "I'm stupefied by the way the Russians receive me, and I hate their wacky system. Why is it the same across all these radically different settings? I think it's because of Haiti. I think it's because I serve the poor. *Love, ID.*"

I had the impression he was angry, disappointed, and a little hurt. A potent combination. And then he went back to work, and I lay in bed trying to read, and in a little while he said, "Whatchya thinkin' over there?" and I felt I was forgiven, and though I wasn't sure for what, this was a relief. It didn't last.

When we got to the airport and learned our flight back to Miami was delayed five hours, we went to a little restaurant on the premises, and Farmer settled in, opening his computer. He called in Spanish to the waitress behind the counter, "Dear lady?" She had her back to us. Without turning, she replied, *"Dígame, mi amor"*—"Speak to me, my love." Farmer laughed. He said to me, "You have to love a country where people do that."

The flight delay hadn't fazed him. In fact, I was thinking, he was apt to be most cheerful when facing adversities, small ones anyway. Then, all of a sudden, he said to me, "If you're going to write about Che, it should be your own opinion. Not mine."

"Why is that?" I asked.

"You now know more about his exhumation than ninety-nine percent of Americans. And also how the Cubans feel about him. The man who dug him up was practically in tears." He was giving me the stare.

"I may be sentimental," he went on, "but I'm not a goofball. I'm a hard-bitten, clinic-building, MDR-treating mother." Then, it seemed, he got to the heart of the matter: what I was going to write about Cuba, especially about him in Cuba.

"When others write about people who live on the edge, who challenge their comfortable lives—and it has happened to me—they usually do it in a way that allows a reader a way out. You could render generosity into pathology, commitment into obsession. That's all in the repertory of someone who wants to put the reader at ease rather than conveying the truth in a compelling manner. I want people to feel unhappy about Lazarus and all the others who are shafted. Otherwise why would I have you with me? I don't have a lot at stake in how you depict me. I've been yelled at by generals and denounced by people who don't have any data when I have a shitload. It does no harm to me, but plenty to my patients. If the very warm reception of me in Cuba is portrayed as because I'm thought to be a sycophantic ally of Cuba, then the Cuban doctors' concern for the poor of Haiti would be lost."

He went on in this way for a time. "If I say that Santiago de las Vegas looks like a nice hacienda with a lot of labs and medical facilities, I'm a tool of the Cuban oppressors." He took up the cause of Dr. Pérez: "Jorge is chief doctor of the Infectious Disease Institute, director of the sanatorium, chair of the national AIDS program, visiting professor in many countries, on the board of directors, by fiat, mine, of our program at Harvard. He has the ear of the president and the minister of health. He's at the pinnacle of power in Cuban medicine and he lives like a lower-middle-class American, and he doesn't care. I have no generic liking for modest living. What I like is that Jorge believes this is right. He doesn't like social inequality. He believes in social justice medicine. That moves me. I hate to see that ridiculed. I hate it."

There was vehemence in his voice, and I felt I was its object, as if I had already ridiculed Dr. Pérez. I'm sure I felt offended, and maybe I felt hurt—though I'd hardly have admitted this at the moment. Farmer's emotional side lay close to the surface, and, as Ophelia said, his emotions were usually sympathetic. He cried openly over patients, and the memories of patients. He greeted everyone in his wide circle with blushing elation. I was no less immune than most people to his warmth. Now he seemed to be withdrawing it, and I felt the chill. Was he saying he'd rather not travel with me anymore? Well, then, the feeling was mutual. This guy kept the cybernetic equivalent of a bumper sticker on his computer, a screen saver that read, "Seek Justice." For me, at the moment, suddenly, the tone of this expressed all my problems with him.

He began to talk about our next destination, Russia. He said it wasn't as important as Haiti.

"Well, do you think I shouldn't come along with you?" I said. I tried to make my tone nonchalant. I'm not sure I succeeded.

He looked surprised. "No, no. It's important."

The scolding, if that's what it was, ended then. He said our conversation had just been the "dismount" of our time in Cuba. The term was one the Farmer family had borrowed from Olympic gymnastics, which they'd watched together on TV on the boat, his buxom sister Peggy throwing out her chest in imitation of the stance the diminutive female athletes would take when they finished their routines. All the interns, residents, and fellows who worked with Farmer at the Brigham knew the term. "Okay, let's do the dismount," he would say, and they'd begin wrapping up discussion of a case.

It was hard to stay angry at Farmer, especially then, as he sat there in his rumpled black suit, waiting out another airport delay in a barren little restaurant, worrying that his admiration for Cuba might be used against his cause and end up harming his patients in the central plateau. I wasn't sure we really had much of an argument over Cuba. Years of bad publicity heaped on the country's government had certainly colored my view of the place but, more than that, had made me wary of coming to conclusions. No question but that Cuba had pulled off something difficult and, in the view from Haiti, enviable—first-rate public health, equitably distributed, in spite of severely limited resources. I just wondered what price in political freedom its people paid for that achievement. But I understood that Farmer would frame the question differently, and ask what price most people would be willing to pay for freedom from illness and premature death. For me, Cuba posed a rather abstract question. For Farmer, it represented hope, proof that a poor country could achieve good public health. "If I could turn Haiti into Cuba, I'd do it in a minute," he had said rather heatedly a while ago. I'd have agreed, if I hadn't felt that the heat was directed at me.

We lingered in the restaurant. I asked him what his hopes for Haiti were.

"I don't have any that are based on analysis or numbers or hardheaded interpretation of the best available data," he said. "But I have hopes for Haiti." These lay partly outside Haiti. "Some people would say things will get so bad that Haitians will revolt. But you can't revolt when you're coughing out your lungs or starving. Someone's going to have to revolt on the Haitians' behalf, including people from the wealthy classes." He added, "But that would be regarded as a total joke by the left."

He turned and gazed out the window. A large sign was affixed to an airplane hangar across the tarmac. It read PATRIA ES HUMANIDAD. An internationalist assertion—the only real nation is humanity.

"I think that's so lovely," Farmer said.

"I don't know," I said. "It seems like a slogan to me."

He looked away. "I guess you're right."

I felt as though I'd punched him. Among a coward's weapons, cynicism is the nastiest of all. "No, it is lovely," I muttered. "If it's really meant."

We got to Miami so late, and he had so much shopping to do, and so many e-mails had accumulated in his account—about a thousand in all, at least two dozen of which concerned patients and required immediate answers—that we almost missed our night flight to Paris. They closed the gate behind us, and Farmer declared our timing "perfect." But the plane was full, and there was no room left for our briefcases. I felt as if I wedged myself into my seat, and Farmer's legs were longer than mine.

For the last day and a half, I'd been suffering from diarrhea. Not from the Cuban water, probably from too many *mojitos*. I had resolved not to tell Farmer and remained determined not to, right up until I told him.

We had taken off. He'd ingested a sleeping pill, a fast-acting benzodiazepine, and his eyelids were fluttering. They opened right up, however, when I made my complaint. He looked over at me, his face utterly serious. "From now on," he said, "I want a full report on all of your bowel movements."

I felt greatly reassured, much better already in fact, and the last remnants of my anger at Farmer seeped away.

It still seemed to me that he took a stance all too conveniently impregnable. He embodied a preferential option for the poor. Therefore, any criticism of him amounted to an assault on the already downtrodden people he served. But I knew by now he wasn't simply posing. I felt something about him that I'd later frame to myself this way: He said patients came first, prisoners second, and students third, but this didn't leave out much of humanity. Every sick person seemed to be a potential patient of Farmer's and every healthy person a potential student. In his mind, he was fighting all poverty all the time, an endeavor full of difficulties and inevitable failures. For him, the reward was inward clarity, and the price perpetual anger or, at best, discomfort with the world, not always on the surface but always there. Sensing this, I'd begun to be relieved of the shallower discomforts I sometimes felt in his company, that I'd felt keenly back in the airport in Cuba. Farmer wasn't put on earth to make anyone feel comfortable, except for those lucky enough to be his patients, and for the moment I had become one of those.

CHAPTER 22

Farmer had loved Paris as a boy from Jenkins Creek on his college semester abroad, and he'd felt great anticipation when he'd taken his wife, Didi, there. It was her first trip ever away from Haiti. Wasn't this the loveliest city in the world? he'd asked her. But the sights of its gorgeous parks and buildings had moved her differently: "Knowing that this splendor came from the suffering of my ancestors." Didi was studying that subject now in Paris, in the archives of the French slave masters, in the detailed records they had kept of their commerce in West Africans. Since then, some of the city's charm had worn off for Farmer.

The sleeping pills that he brought to get us through the flights have left my memories of our stop in Paris all wrapped up in gauze. I recall an early morning, Farmer gazing out the windows of the cab, reentering the first world by staring at the cardboard box–like high-rises of the periphery, where, he said, many of the indigent of Paris had been relocated. As we entered the city proper, that great dove-colored epicurean city, he murmured something about how much could be done in Haiti if only he could get his hands on the money that the first world spent on pet grooming.

The cab let us off in the Marais district, a place of narrow streets and sidewalks, of bistros, diminutive hotels, and shops. The Farmer family residence was an apartment of three small rooms, borrowed from one of his oldest friends from Duke. Didi—tall and stately—met us at the door with an enormous smile. I remember thinking that Didi probably *was* the most beautiful woman from Cange. And I remember Farmer in his black suit, dancing with his daughter, holding her to his chest, swaying from side to side in a loopy, long-limbed waltz. And the little girl's dark eyes, which her face hadn't yet grown into, fixed in serious rapture on some invisible object on the ceiling. Later, Farmer sat on the sofa and watched Catherine play with her stuffed animals. Didi called to him from the kitchen. When did he leave for Moscow?

Tomorrow morning, Farmer said.

From the kitchen came the sound of something dropping and a deep-throated exclamation.

I looked over at Farmer. He was clasping his knees with his elbows and covering his mouth with both hands. I remember thinking, despite my enveloping haze, I'd remember this. It was the first time I'd seen him at a loss for words or action.

Ironic, I suppose, that just when his organization's endeavors had ceased to be global in theory and had become global in fact, a child had entered his life. Lately, he received a fair amount of criticism from friends for not spending more time with his family, and there were some who, when they spoke about this matter out of his earshot, seemed oddly animated. Their voices would rise, or they would smile conspiratorially. "Can you imagine what it's like being married to him?" I wonder if this was a species of moral envy. Jim Kim said, "Paul has a gift for making people feel guilty." Farmer counseled others to take vacations while taking none himself. He didn't disapprove of others having luxuries, so long as they gave something to the causes of the poor. He demanded a great deal from protégés and colleagues, and he always forgave them when they didn't measure up. And so I think it was a relief, for some, to find what looked like a chink in his moral armor.

In Haiti, we'd had a conversation about his daughter. A month after she was born, a woman had come to Zanmi Lasante suffering from eclampsia. It is a disease of pregnancy, of mysterious origin, found preponderantly among poor women. It leads to protein in the urine, hypertension, seizures, and sometimes death, for both mother and child. The treatment is magnesium sulfate and delivery of the child. The clinic was very busy. Farmer was rushing around trying to get the treatment started. He was saying to the staff, "Come on, get off your butts. Get an IV in, I want to induce her now." The baby was alive. He could hear the heartbeat.

He remembered, "The mother was seizing. I said, 'Hurry!' Everything was going okay. Then the baby was born, and it was dead. A full-term, beautiful baby, and I started to weep. I had to excuse myself and go outside. I wondered, What's going on? Then I realized I was crying because of Catherine." He had imagined her in the place of the still-born child. "So you love your own child more than these kids," he said to himself.

He went on: "I thought I was the king of empathy for these poor kids, but if I was the king of empathy, why this big shift because of my daughter? It was a failure of empathy, the inability to love other children as much as yours. The thing is, everybody understands that, encourages that, praises you for it. But the hard thing is the other."

I thought about this for a while, attempting to frame my question delicately. Finally, I just tried to disassociate myself from it: "Some people would say, Where do you get off thinking you're different from everyone and can love the children of others as much as your own. What would you say to that?"

"Look," he replied. "All the great religious traditions of the world say, Love thy neighbor as thyself. My answer is, I'm sorry, I can't, but I'm gonna keep on trying, *comma.*"

I imagine that many people would like to construct a life like Farmer's, to wake up knowing what they ought to do and feeling that they were doing it. But I can't think that many would willingly take on the difficulties, giving up their comforts and time with family. It wasn't as if this stopover in Paris represented all there was to his domestic life. He and Didi and Catherine spent the summers together in Cange, and no doubt those periods would lengthen once Didi finished her studies. But his days and nights looked hard and in some ways lonesome. He was carrying a pair of photographs on this light month for travel. One was of Catherine, and at each stop he'd show it off to friends like any proud parent, but then sometimes he'd show the other, a photo of a Haitian child of about the same age, except in the throes of kwashiorkor. At first, this seemed perverse to me. But the other, starving child wasn't an abstraction, like the pictures of starving children on TV. She was Farmer's patient, and I think in his mind she stood for all the others, including tuberculous prisoners in Russia, for whom he was leaving his daughter tomorrow on the morning flight to Moscow. I don't think anyone who knew how much Farmer craved connections among all parts of his life could have looked at him at that moment on the couch in Paris, all folded up as if trying to hide, and not felt some sympathy for his predicament.

The moment passed. Farmer was stopping in Paris mainly for Catherine's second birthday party. The event was a success, and Catherine clapped her hands at her present—a mechanical bird on a wire that flew around the small living room. He'd bought it in the Miami airport. It was one of the reasons we'd almost missed the plane to Paris. Among the guests, there were a couple of members of the French family for whom Farmer had worked as an au pair, almost twenty years ago, during his student year abroad. These days they did some fund-raising for PIH. There were also Haitian friends at the party, in France long enough that they no longer passed what Farmer called "the fat test"—that is, they looked well-fed—but Haiti was almost all they talked about. There was a family friend from Burkina Faso, who told me he was homesick, and I was reminded of something Farmer had said, that PIH headquarters wasn't Boston or even Haiti but wherever PIH-ers happened to be. He had built a web of acquaintance as large as any major politician's. The difference was that not many people in his web remained mere acquaintances for long, and not many would have found it easy simply to slip away, even if they wanted to. For Farmer, the worst kind of exile wouldn't be geographical. It would be something like excommunication.

Before he went to bed, he phoned his mother in Florida, to ask her to give him a wake-up call at 7:00 A.M. here in Paris. Didi shook her head. "We have an alarm clock," she said to me, but she was smiling.

I counted time zones. His mother would have to be up at 1:00 A.M. to make the call. I wondered if she minded, but she told me some months later, "I just think it's so cool that at forty he still does that. I'd miss it if he didn't."

＝

We got to the airport early, for once, and went to a café for breakfast. "Okay," Farmer said, when we found a table, "time to get to work." He pulled out his most recent *bwat* list. Only about two-thirds of the little boxes had been checked. "This is shameful." He stared at the sheets of paper. "All these *bwats* were supposed to be done before we left Cuba."

Among them was a dual *bwat,* one that consisted of two chores; if he completed either, he'd get to check the box. The dual *bwat* commanded him either to buy new underwear or to finish a letter. "I didn't get the underwear, so . . ." This was a letter he had started during a hike we'd taken back in Haiti. He pulled the unfinished page from his briefcase. It had a grease stain on it, from some article of the fifth food group he'd eaten on the hike. "It seems fitting to write you as I sit in the middle of the Haitian countryside," the letter began. He bent over it, writing on.

"Is this *bwat* transfer or *bwat* cheating?" I asked.

"Depends on whether or not you have an H of G for the endeavor," he said, without looking up.

"An H of G" was short for "a hermeneutic of generosity," which he had defined once for me in an e-mail: "I have a hermeneutic of generosity for you because I know you're a good guy. Therefore I will interpret what you say and do in a favorable light. Seems like I'm the one who should hope for as much from you." I have counted scores of terms like that one in his lexicon, which was also the lexicon of PIH. Jim and Ophelia had invented some, and some came from the Brigham, but most were Farmer's, or his family's.

One time his brother Jeff, the wrestler, sent him a card in which he misspelled the word "Haitians." He spelled it "Hatians." So in PIH lingo, Haitians were "Hat-eans" or simply "Hats," and their country was "Hatland." The French were "Fran-chayze," their tongue "Fran-chayze language," and Russians were "Rooskies." A "chatterjee" was a person of East Indian descent—there were a few in PIH—who talked a lot. Farmer referred to himself as "white trash"—he had an old photo to prove it, his extended family at a picnic around a couch outdoors. The man who railed about the plight of impoverished women every-where would in private, poking fun, employ terms like "chicks." "I don't care about any of that stuff," he told me once. "Just the one thing." Impolite terms, used intramurally, were meant as philosophi-cal rebukes to the misplaced preoccupations of those who believed in "identity politics," in the idea that all members of an oppressed mi-nority were equally oppressed, which all too conveniently obscured the fact that there were real differences in the "shaftedness," also sometimes called the "degrees of hose-edness," that people of the same race or gender suffered. "All suffering isn't equal" was an article of the PIH faith, generated in reaction to the many times when they had tried to raise money and instead had been offered lectures about the universality of suffering, or simply lines like "The rich have prob-lems, too." (Farmer once taught a course at Harvard called Varieties of Human Suffering.)

"When people get around Paul, they start talking like Paul," his old friend from medical school the writer Ethan Canin said. "He's such a word gymnast." There was an obvious utility in the brevity of terms like "H of G," for a mind moving fast, and for people trying to keep up. When, for instance, "TBMI" (transnational bureaucrats managing inequality) produced clever arguments (also known as "well-formed stool") against treating MDR or AIDS, one could simply say, "Love, ID," and be completely understood. Everyone in PIH knew that "DQ" stood for "Drama Queen," and a DQ proposal meant an emotional appeal. ("We could use a DQ quote here, and a generic inequality-of-outcomes over here," I once heard Farmer say to a young assistant working with him on a speech.) "Geek flowers" was the completed research that PIH-ers presented to Farmer or Kim, and "scholbutt" was short for "scholarly buttressing," which meant that every statement of fact Farmer made in a paper had to be verified as coming from some au-thoritative source. ("He's neurotic about having it all perfect," said a medical student who did a lot of scholbutt for Farmer. ("Not because he's anal but because when you're doing these things for the poor, amidst arguments that it's not cost-effective to treat them, you have to be perfect or you'll be picked apart.")

"Lugar" was luggage. "Koutoums" meant "customs." To commit "a seven-three" was to use seven words where three would do, and a "ninety-nine one hundred" was quitting on a nearly completed job. ("Nothing pisses me off like a ninety-nine one hundred," Farmer would say.) PIH-ers often said "Thank you" to people who had done something for a third party, for anyone who belonged to the multitudinous group known variously as "the indigent sick," "the shafted," and "the poor," the last being the term of choice in PIH because, as Farmer would say, it was the term that most Haitians used to describe themselves.

You could hang around the inner circle of PIH for a long time without understanding what the rules were and feeling excluded, and the more left out you felt, the more you suspected you were being told you weren't as good as they were, even as you suspected that your irritation proved it. To me, the inner circle of PIH seemed like a club, or even like a family, which was deeply opposed to the concept of insiders and outsiders, and yet equipped with its own special bylaws and language. Say that to Farmer and he'd reply, "If so, it's surely the most inclusive damn club in the world, being full of people with AIDS, WL's galore, tons of students, church ladies, lots of patients, and it's a club that grows and never shrinks." And Farmer had a way of creating a club that consisted just of him and you.

Back in Haiti, he had established a piece of private language for our month of travel. Discussing malaria with me, he'd explained there were four types, only one of which, falciparum, was often fatal. "So which one do you suppose Haiti has?" he asked. Then he added, "*But it's not drug-resistant, the way it is in Africa.*" He smiled, and then, adapting his favorite line from the movie *Caddyshack*, he said, "So we got dat goin' for us." Then he pointed at me, and I soon learned this meant I was supposed to utter the next line in the movie: "Which is nice." After I got the hang of this call and response, I enjoyed it. And I must confess I felt a certain pleasure now, at the airport café, in knowing what he meant by "an H of G."

He went on writing his letter. I looked around. The airport, Charles de Gaulle, has an angular, steel-and-glass simplicity, which struck me just then as frighteningly complex, which made me feel projected into a future I didn't understand. I thought of its duty-free shop, where one could buy first-class pâté, *confit d'oie, grand cru* wines. "You started that letter on a hike in rural Haiti," I mused aloud, thinking now of those arid highlands, of medieval peasant huts, donkey ambulances. "It seems like another world."

Farmer looked up, smiling, and in a chirpy-sounding voice he said, "But that feeling has the disadvantage of being . . ." He paused a beat. "Wrong."

"Well," I retorted, "it depends on how you look at it."

"No, it doesn't," he replied, in a very pleasant voice. "The polite thing to say would be, 'You're right. It's a parallel universe. There really is no relation between the massive accumulation of wealth in one part of the world and abject misery in another.' " He looked at me. He'd made me laugh. "You know I'm being funny about something serious," he said.

One time I listened to Farmer give a talk on HIV to a class at the Harvard School of Public Health, and in the midst of reciting data, he mentioned the Haitian phrase "looking for life, destroying life." Then he explained, "It's an expression Haitians use if a poor woman selling mangoes falls off a truck and dies." I felt as if for that moment I could see a little way into his mind. It seemed like a place of hyperconnectivity. At moments like that, I thought that what he wanted was to erase both time and geography, connecting all parts of his life and tying them instrumentally to a world in which he saw intimate, inescapable connections between the gleaming corporate offices of Paris and New York and a legless man lying on the mud floor of a hut in the remotest part of remote Haiti. Of all the world's errors, he seemed to feel, the most fundamental was the "erasing" of people, the "hiding away" of suffering. "My big struggle is how people can not care, erase, not remember."

I had wondered if there was room in his philosophy for anyone but the world's poor and people who campaigned on behalf of the poor. One day on an airplane, he confided to me that he thought of all our fellow passengers as patients. An attendant's voice had said over the intercom, "Is there a doctor onboard?" He'd gotten up at once and ministered to a middle-aged, evidently middle-class American man who, as it turned out, wasn't having a heart attack. Back in his seat afterward, Farmer said this happened to him about once in every eighteen flights. I had the impression that he wouldn't have minded if it happened every flight.

Embracing a continuity and interconnectedness that excluded no one seemed like another of Farmer's peculiar liberties. It came with a lot of burdens, of course, but it also freed him from the efforts that many people make to find refuge and distinction from their pasts, and from the mass of their fellow human beings.

CHAPTER 23

The World Bank was planning a loan to try to stanch the TB epidemic in Russia. Farmer was going to Moscow, for the fifth time now, to work on the terms of the loan. On the airplane, he explained the history of this mission.

About two years back, Howard Hiatt had sent him to the Open Society Institute, George Soros's foundation, to search for new money to sustain the project in Peru. The OSI declined to get involved, but said in a letter that they understood the importance of PIH's project because they were doing similar work in Russia. They described this in some detail.

Farmer remembered that he read the letter on his way to a meeting and that it made him stop on the sidewalk: "Holy shit!" He was already aware that Soros had put up about $13 million for TB pilot projects in Russia, but he hadn't known the details until then. They would use only the DOTS strategy. They would treat all patients for nonresistant TB, and for those who didn't get better, they'd provide hospice care to ease their deaths. But the collapse of the Soviet Union had created ideal ingredients both for a very large epidemic and for rampant drug resistance within it: a failing TB control system had led to many uncompleted therapies; rising crime had led to overcrowded prisons.

With Hiatt's blessing, Farmer wrote the foundation's director a courtly two-page letter, explaining that their project was bound to fail. He ended up in George Soros's Manhattan office. Farmer made his case. Then Soros ordered that the director of his Russian TB program, Alex Goldfarb, the Russian émigré and microbiologist, be contacted at once. Soros yelled at Goldfarb for a while over the phone. Then he asked Farmer to help fix the Russian pilot projects.

Farmer wavered briefly. At the time, he still had to travel fairly often to Peru. Russia would mean even more days and weeks away from Haiti, a place much more afflicted by TB and every other disease. Still, PIH could legitimately use some of Soros's money to pay salaries. Besides, Russia's epidemic was ravaging its prisons, and prisoners were part of PIH's special constituency—the Gospels said so; you could look it up, in Matthew 25. And Russia might represent the kind of opportunity Paul and Jim had hoped for when they'd taken on Peru, a chance to affect health policy toward the poor on a global scale. Russia bordered twelve other countries these days, and those countries bordered some of the world's wealthiest. "It's much more difficult to make arguments for equity in a place like Haiti, which can be so easily hidden away. But it's pretty hard to hide Russia," Farmer reasoned. Russian TB might show the world the consequences of neglecting the health of poor people everywhere, of neglecting Haiti.

So he went on a tour of Siberian prisons with Goldfarb and some other advisers to the Soros Foundation and some Russian officials. Before the trip Goldfarb had referred to Farmer as "the evil enemy from the north." They returned from Siberia as friends. By then Goldfarb understood Farmer better. At one point he'd asked Farmer what fee he charged for his services, and Farmer had said, "Alex, you idiot, what's my *fee*? I charge a lot for prisoners, POWs, and the destitute sick. And I really ramp it up for refugees." Mostly, though, what united them was the spectacle they'd witnessed in the Russian gulag.

In most places, prisoners contract TB at higher rates than civilians. In Russia's prisons, though, the incidence was forty to fifty times higher. Moreover, the majority of sick inmates had strains resistant to at least one drug, while nearly a third in some of the jails had full-fledged MDR. Tuberculosis had become the leading cause of death in the prisons, but not all were dying there. Many inmates were surviving long enough to get released and bring their drug-resistant strains of TB back into civilian society. And when they got out, most of those who were sick didn't get treated, mainly because Russia's huge civilian TB control system was itself in shambles.

The situation was dire, but so far the international response had been puny. About a dozen non-Russian organizations were trying to figure out how to control the epidemic. Most had only small amounts to spend—hundreds of thousands of dollars or a million or two. Their projects, some well-managed, all established in the face of great obstacles, had shown what they hadn't intended—that DOTS alone not only wouldn't serve but would amplify the epidemic. In the Russian oblast of Ivanovo, the U.S. Centers for Disease Control and Prevention had knowingly treated MDR patients with drugs they were resistant to and had cured only 5 percent of them. And Farmer predicted—correctly as it would turn out—that many of that 5 percent would relapse. Even Doctors Without Borders, praised by the Nobel Prize Committee for its work on TB in Russia, had so far hewed to the code of DOTS alone, and had cured only 46 percent of the patients they'd treated in Prison Colony 33 in Kemerovo. "Managerial successes, clinical failures" Farmer called these efforts in a paper.

The epidemic he'd seen in Siberia's prisons was worse than anything he'd seen in Peru, and in some respects anything he'd witnessed in Haiti. So when they got back to Moscow from their tour of the gulag, he and Goldfarb held a press conference to spread the dire news, but they did so on the day when, in Washington, the special prosecutor released his report on the Monica Lewinsky scandal. Only a handful of reporters came.

Farmer and Goldfarb flew on to New York, for an "emergency meeting" with Soros. For Farmer, meetings with the man were often refreshing. Farmer once made a quick estimate of what it would cost to control TB throughout the world—about $5 billion, he thought. He mentioned this figure to public health people, and they said such a sum could never be raised. When Soros saw the estimate, though, he said, "Is that all? You only need that?" In New York, Farmer and Goldfarb asked Soros to put up more money at once for treating TB in Russia. Soros said that would just delay the international response. Instead, among other things, he arranged a meeting at the White House, his friend Hillary Clinton presiding. Farmer and Goldfarb wrote the talking points for Soros and critiqued the ones prepared for the First Lady.

The upshot wasn't all Farmer thought it should be. He'd hoped for large grants from foundations and wealthy nations. Instead, Hillary Clinton prevailed on the World Bank to look into giving Russia a loan. And the World Bank created something called a mission to Moscow, a group of economists, epidemiologists, and public health experts who would work out the details of a loan.

Predictably, Farmer got more and more deeply involved, bringing the rest of PIH along. The whole crew labored on a report commissioned by Soros—and in seven months turned out a book with 177 pages of text, 115 pages of appendices, 976 references, with chapters describing the problem of MDR in Russia, Azerbaijan, Peru, and South Africa, and a final chapter about how to create a proper treatment program. It stirred up some press, and WHO endorsed the volume by contributing an introduction. Farmer also agreed to serve as the chief but unpaid consultant on TB in Russian prisons for the World Bank's mission to Moscow—unpaid at his insistence; he deplored some of the bank's policies; Soros was taking care of his expenses.

=====

We arrived in Moscow late in the afternoon. Most of the passengers got up from their seats before the plane had reached the gate, and the flight attendant pleaded uselessly over the intercom, "Would you please remain seated?"

Farmer looked around the cabin. "I have a soft spot for the Rooskies. They get up when they feel like it. Of course, the Russians have been used like furniture for the last four hundred years. No wonder they want to stand."

Farmer believed, obviously, in the importance of intentions and the power of will, but also in revelation, in "signs." Today, it seemed to me, not all omens were good. Inside Moscow's main airport, which had all the charm of a warehouse, we filled out the wrong entry forms, and for the first time since I'd been traveling with Farmer, I witnessed his friendliness fail with a stranger. He smiled at the grim-faced, uniformed woman at customs and said, "Sorry. Next time I'll learn Russian."

"Next time fill out the English form," she snarled.

But she let us pass. Farmer said, with sympathy, not irony, "That's all right. After all, she's an employee of a defeated superpower."

Outside, the afternoon sun was an orange sliver on an icy horizon.

In the morning, outside our hotel, the air steamed from mouths— of pedestrians, of grates in the street. From the hotel's front windows, you could look across a broad avenue at the Kremlin Palace, crenellated towers on high walls, all in perfect repair, stretching out of sight. Beyond, I could see the onion-topped towers of St. Basil's Cathedral. Farmer had said he thought it one of the world's most beautiful buildings, but marred by the fact that it had been built to celebrate Ivan the Terrible's bloody victory over the Tartars. Erasing history, he liked to say, always served the interests of power. Anyway, I knew I wouldn't be going to the cathedral with him. In Moscow, we were going to practice his kind of tourism, a transit one could make in any major city in the world. We—Farmer and I and Alex Goldfarb, who had flown in from New York—were going to visit a prison.

═══

Moscow's Central Prison, Matrosskaya Tishina, was the city's largest jail, designated a *sizo,* a detention center. The building was immense, though I couldn't grasp its actual dimensions because of the complexity of turnings, through doorways where you had to duck your head, and climbings, up ancient metal staircases, and hikes, down corridors that made me think of abandoned subway tunnels, with some sort of yellow fiberboard slapped haphazardly on the walls. "In summer," Farmer whispered to me, "the air-conditioning doesn't work so well." He added, "The last few years I've been doing my practicum in comparative penology." We passed through various climate zones, from warm to cold to warm again, and regions of odor, some of food, others hard to place—it seemed better not to know.

"Don't get lost," a prison official said. "This is not a good place to get lost."

We passed a file of inmates, all dressed in baggy pants, in ragged coats and caps, gray faces in dim light; one had the crookedest nose I'd ever seen. Then we reached the prison hospital. "Think of Cuba," Farmer whispered to me. "Look at this shitty place." Our guides were doctors in olive drab uniforms and public health officials in olive drab uniforms, and they themselves deplored the conditions. They opened the door to a cell reserved for patients with AIDS. "There are fewer than in the usual cells," one of the female doctors said.

"How many?"

"Only fifty in this room."

Farmer went in first, followed by a translator. It was a dingy gray chamber, smaller than many American living rooms, full of double-decker beds, laundry hanging from clotheslines. Most of the men were young. Their faces looked gray, but perhaps that was because of the dimness of the light. In a moment Farmer was shaking hands with them, touching arms and shoulders, and in another moment loud voices all around him were competing to air grievances. "You should go to the courts and stand up for the rights of the AIDS-infected on trial," said one of the inmates.

"Tell him I do that in the U.S.," Farmer said to the translator. "But since I'm not a Russian citizen . . ."

One prisoner, older than the rest, evidently something like a spokes-man, declared that he had merely been a witness to the killing of a man, but because he had AIDS he got a sentence of five years. The actual killer, who was tried with him, got only three. "And when I get out, I will cut his head off," he said. Everyone, prisoners and doc-tors, laughed, a deafening sound in the cramped cell. Farmer made a note—"AIDS patients get longer prison sentences?"—and said he'd pass it on to the World Bank's AIDS specialist.

He thanked the prisoners. The spokesman said, "I wish you would come more often."

"I would like to."

We left the cell of the fifty AIDS patients, and the door clanged shut behind us. That sound, of heavy old metal on metal, echoing down a dimly lit hallway. I couldn't see the end of the hallway. I couldn't hear the end of the echo. "Ever imagine what it would be like to hear that sound on the other side of the door?" I asked Farmer.

"Every time," he said.

It really wasn't hard to imagine—making the kind of mistake that would end in a cell inside this place. In Russia just now, a young man could get thrown in jail for stealing a loaf of bread or a bottle of vodka and, because the criminal justice system was clogged, languish in a detention center for a year or even four years before his case came to trial. While waiting or while serving his sentence, he'd probably get infected with TB—it was estimated that about 80 percent of all Russian prisoners had bacilli in their bodies. Once infected, he stood a better than average chance of coming down with the active disease—because of poor hygiene, inadequate nutrition, the prevalence of other illnesses in jail. And the underfinanced prison medical service didn't have the equipment or drugs to achieve a respectable cure rate even among the inmates with drug-susceptible TB. A young prisoner could contract susceptible TB and, through inadequate treatment, end up with MDR. Or, increasingly likely, he could catch a strain of MDR directly from another inmate and die from it before he even got sentenced for stealing his loaf of bread.

We were led on another twisty passage, down a winding metal stair, then through what looked like a medieval dungeon. We passed an old man pushing a cart. It had big metal cans on it. An enormous ladle stuck out of one. He stopped at a hole in a cell door. A face appeared at the hole. "The food's pretty good actually," Farmer said to me. "Salty." High praise from the doctor with high blood pressure.

We arrived at the TB department. "The doctors are overworked and have almost no protection," a prison official said. "The X-ray equipment it is exhausted. There are not enough drugs for the patients that we have. We do not have laboratory support from Moscow."

They weren't sure how many prisoners had drug-resistant strains. Certainly more than a handful. Of 100,000 inmates sick with TB, perhaps 30,000 had MDR. Last October, Farmer had appeared on the TV show *60 Minutes* to talk about the epidemic in Russia and its former republics. "We're going to have to declare this a global public health emergency," he had said.

"How much time is there before this gets really out of hand?" the TV host had asked.

"I think it's already out of hand," Farmer had replied.

We lingered in the hall of the TB department. One of the Russian doctors said, "We get no information from the other institutions where the prisoners come from. This is a division of the railway station. Fifty percent are not from Moscow."

Farmer asked how long it took for a tuberculous inmate to get from here to a Siberian prison.

"About a month. They are sent to way stations. There is no way to maintain treatment en route."

Farmer turned to Goldfarb and said in a low voice, "These prisoner transfers are going to be nightmares."

We went into another cell, this one filled with TB patients, a cell much the same as the last but a little more crowded and humid—the humidity that comes from many pairs of lungs exhaling. Several men were coughing, each distinctively, I thought—a Chaliapin bass, a baritone, a tenor. Farmer stood beside a bed, his arm resting on the mattress of an upper berth. "You look good," he said to one of the men. "Anybody coughing up blood?"

"No."

"So pretty much people are getting better?"

"It's not worse," said a prisoner.

He asked them where they came from. Grozny, Volga, Baku. "Tell them I've been to Baku," Farmer said to the translator. "And it's better to be here. Tell them I've been to Colony Three."

A young man sitting on an upper berth said, "I saw you in Colony Three. You were with a woman."

"Yes, I was there with a woman!" Farmer exclaimed. He reached out his hand and shook with the man. "It's nice to see you again."

It was time to leave. "Good luck," said Farmer through the translator. "Tell them I hope everybody gets better."

We headed back toward the prison office. "I like these prison medical people," Farmer said to me. "They're trying." He turned to the translator. "Tell Ludmilla"—she was one of the Russian doctors—"I've met some extremely dedicated prison doctors." He had singled out Ludmilla because she'd told him a story about an Italian human rights activist who had inspected the prison and accused her of mistreating AIDS patients by keeping them isolated from the other inmates. Farmer had said, "In a setting where there's a lot of TB? *Not* to isolate them would be a violation of human rights!"

Farmer spoke softly to me as we walked along. "They have seven hundred hospital beds in this place, and about five hundred are filled with TB patients. That's a clue, just a *clue* that there might be a problem." On top of drug resistance—one of the doctors had told Farmer—the incidence of syphilis was rising. Alarming, because rising syphilis announces the imminence of AIDS, which would grossly magnify the TB epidemic. "It's gonna be a fucking disaster," Farmer was saying, as the hosts ushered us into the central office, a mustard-colored chamber.

Now the crude conference table there was laid with a feast. Farmer declared, "Oh, thank you! Just what I like!" He murmured to me, "I was afraid of this. I hate vodka." But he sat down and knocked it back with expertly feigned pleasure, just as he did in Haiti when eating from the fifth food group. Toasts were offered, and countertoasts. After a while, Farmer's grew lengthy.

"I have been working in Haiti for almost twenty years, ever since I was a young chap, and some years ago I was asked by the state of Massachusetts to be a TB commissioner, and I said, 'What the hell do we do?' I was in Haiti and I had a couple of MDR-TB patients and I took sputums and I brought them to Boston. And I took them into the lab and I wrote, 'Paul Farmer, State TB Commissioner.' I wanted them to process my samples from Haiti and they did and never asked any questions, so I did it more and more and then I did it with sputums from Peru, and of course, eventually they asked me why. I said, 'Massachusetts is a great state, it has a *big* TB lab, *lots* of TB doctors, *lots* of TB nurses, *lots* of TB lab specialists. It lacks only one thing. Tuberculosis.' "

The chief of the Russian doctors—a colonel—laughed. A woman doctor said gravely, "We have lots of TB and no labs."

More toasts, more vodka. The colonel reached in his pocket, began to take a pack of cigarettes from it, then paused and asked Farmer, "Is America a democracy?"

Paul's face grew serious. "I think whenever a people has enormous resources, it is easy for them to call themselves democratic. I think of myself more as a physician than as an American. Ludmilla and I, we belong to the nation of those who care for the sick. Americans are lazy democrats, and it is my belief, as someone who shares the same nationality as Ludmilla, I think that the rich can always call themselves democratic, but the sick people are not among the rich." I thought he was done, but he was only pausing for the interpreter to catch up. "Look, I'm very proud to be an American. I have many opportunities because I'm American. I can travel freely throughout the world, I can start projects, but that's called privilege, not democracy."

As Farmer had talked, the colonel's face had begun showing signs of exertion. Now he let his laughter out. He said, "But I only wanted to know if you would permit me to smoke a cigarette."

Goldfarb made a face. "Paul. He wanted to know if he could smoke, and you gave heem a speech on socialism and democracy."

"But the speech was marvelous," said the colonel, smiling at Farmer, who seemed on the verge of falling asleep.

Goldfarb turned to the colonel. "Tomorrow Paul will represent your interests at the World Bank."

Farmer shook himself alert. "The only thing wrong, I don't think it should be a loan. But for the international community of healers it will be a good thing. I pray"—he put his hands together in a steeple—"that it will go well."

=

In the world of TB control, experts were still wrangling about MDR treatment, a fray in which journal articles were the principal weapons. But, as Howard Hiatt said, Farmer and Kim had shown that MDR could be treated, and indeed cost-effectively. Partly thanks to the example of their work in Peru, the World Bank shared a consensus: the loan should be used to treat all strains of TB in Russia; that is, should be used for both DOTS and DOTS-plus campaigns. The Russian officials agreed; in fact, this had long been their essential position. But opinions still divided on how the loan would be allocated. And the mixture of players involved in the discussions seemed combustible, like the nations of Europe before World War I—a stew of World Bank consultants with substantial résumés, some with egos to match, combined with Russian colonels and generals and former apparatchiks and old TB warriors, members of a defeated empire, on the lookout for condescension.

Alex Goldfarb was himself part of the complexity.

One night over cocktails, one of the members of the World Bank team had said to Farmer, "I like Alex, but please keep him away from the meetings." Goldfarb was Farmer's main ally in the negotiations, Farmer representing the bank on the problem of TB among prisoners and Goldfarb representing the Russian Ministry of Justice, which ran the prisons. For Farmer and Goldfarb, the objective this week was to make sure that the prisons got a fair share of the loan. Farmer had told me that he had an additional task: "I have to keep Alex in check."

Most mornings and evenings during the week in Moscow, Alex came to our hotel to discuss strategy. He looked professorial, with his beard, his slight stoop, his tweed and corduroy. "I am very respected biochemist," he told me.

Farmer turned to me. "He discovered one of the genes that creates resistance." He smiled at Alex. "Otherwise he's not much."

Then Farmer began to give Alex a rundown of the meetings so far.

Alex listened for a time, then said, speaking of Farmer's chief antagonist on the World Bank team, "Who is this asshole? I am so amazed by him. Such arrogance and such ignorance. Why don't I put this story in *Izvestia* tomorrow?"

"I knew you would say that," said Farmer. He looked at me. "You laugh, but he does things like that."

Alex went on, "The World Bank brought here an expert with a turban from India, in this terrible snow, and he doesn't know anything about Russia, and he's feenished. These people don't know what is going on with this country."

Farmer tried to continue. Alex broke in. Farmer said, "Let me finish."

Alex said, "Let me tell you something. The people whom you are meeting with are totally insigneeficant."

"Alex, would you let me fucking finish?" said Farmer. Across the hotel dining room, heads turned. Farmer lowered his voice. "You don't have to keep interrupting me. You change our proposal the way you want it. My job is to tell you what they're going to gripe about."

"Insigneeficant persons," said Alex.

There were many divisions attached to these meetings, according to Alex. Here was the political landscape, according to him. The foreigners hammering out the details of the loan harbored many animosities. For instance, the World Health Organization bureaucrats stationed in Moscow resented the intrusion on their turf of nongovernmental organizations, such as PIH and Soros's foundation, which itself, according to Alex, contained competing factions, because Soros liked to create competition inside his own organizations. In addition, some of these WHO people were Polish, not Russian, and between the two nationalities old hatreds still endured.

Alex related all this with, I thought, a certain relish. Then he said, "But this is insigneeficant." What mattered, first of all, was the Russian split, between the Ministry of Health and the Ministry of Justice. The Ministry of Health, in charge of the civilian sector, wanted overall control of the loan. Not mainly, Alex said, in order to deal with TB but in order to prop up their crumbling system. There were also shadowy alliances between the Ministry of Health and Russian drug companies, which would not get to supply the vast quantities of TB drugs required if price and quality were the criteria. Moreover, the Ministry of Health bureaucrats felt insulted by many of the internationalists—among others, by Alex, as Farmer pointed out. Alex had called them clowns and worse.

As for the Ministry of Justice, Alex went on, its motives probably weren't pure, but its intentions were correct. Nearly half of all TB cases and most of the drug-resistant ones languished in the prisons. And the prisons were playing the role of what Alex called "an epidemiological pump," spreading TB among prisoners, then sending them back to civilian society. "This pump is replaced every three years. So the best way to clean society is to purify the prisons, just like you clean oil filter in your car."

Farmer agreed with all this and felt, in addition, that prisoners deserved attention first. "The point is you're exposing prisoners to higher risk, so it's wrong not to treat them first." He believed that Justice sincerely wanted to cure the tuberculous prisoners. Why wouldn't they? The prison epidemic threatened their own personnel, indeed their own empire. He felt they were sincere, in part because Justice had given him free access to all sorts of confidential documents. But at the meeting today, the consensus on the World Bank team had seemed to be that Justice—the prisoners—would get only 20 percent of the loan. It was on the question of how to change this view, how to get Justice 50 percent of the loan, that Farmer and Alex divided.

Farmer sympathized with the Ministry of Health. He had courted the old TB warriors among them, and many liked him. Diplomacy and data and personal charm, he seemed to say, could win over all sides, and unite all factions against the bacillus, their common enemy after all.

In response to this sort of talk, Alex said, "Paul. You are so naïve." It was power and money that would prevail, as always. For the moment, he would let Farmer do things his way. "But there is Plan B. Actually, I like Plan B. We fail. The prisons get shortchanged. All the money goes to the Ministry of Health. Then we raise hell. Then we have a perfect weapon to go raise private money."

Farmer said, "But you won't do that yet, because I'll feel I wasted a whole year in the World Bank offices."

"Why did you go there?" said Alex.

"Why did I go there?" said Farmer, raising his voice. "Because you told me to!"

Alex chuckled. "Of course I did."

For a time, I thought Goldfarb might be right, that the odds were long against Farmer's getting the prisoners half the loan. Farmer had told me on the plane to Moscow that he was tired of the World Bank meetings and the arguments, in conference rooms that grew increasingly airless, where there were no patients, his thoughts straying back to Cange: When the next meningitis victim came in, would one of the doctors, in his absence, do a spinal tap? And he seemed physically exhausted. Our first morning in Moscow, at breakfast—for him, a euphemism for coffee—he told me, "I'm still biologically deranged." He wore his third and last shirt. One of the buttons was missing. His black suit looked as if he'd slept in it. Actually, he hadn't slept. "But I did answer all four hundred and thirteen e-mails," he said, momentarily buoyant.

One quadrant of his hair stuck up like a rooster's, and his face and neck were red, probably because in his mind he was already arguing. Among the e-mails he'd dealt with last night, he'd found one that quoted a member of the World Bank team as saying, "It's ridiculous and too expensive, this proposal for the prisons. It's ridiculous." Now Farmer himself said, over his coffee, "The battle is joined. But this is a ten-year program. This is a very long process. Ten years. I think I should be nonconflictual at least for a day. I'm trying to talk to myself. I'm trying to keep myself from slugging the guy."

He went on, "The prisoners are dying. They'll go on dying." Then he looked at his watch. He was nearly late for the morning meeting. He hurried off, pulling on his overcoat. The cord of his computer trailed out his briefcase, dragging along on the carpet behind him. "Sir," said the doorman, picking up Farmer's gloves.

"Oh, thank you!" said Farmer and eagerly asked, "Is it going to snow?" as the doorman held the door and Farmer hunched his shoulders against the blast of January Moscow air.

In the evening he looked somewhat restored. The head of the Russian negotiating team had held aloft a translated version of an article

Farmer had written called "Resurgent TB in Russia" and had said, "You are the only one who understands TB in Russia." Then the negotiators had wrangled over the preliminary plan Farmer presented for the prisons, especially over the part that would give tuberculous prisoners extra food. Was extra food necessary for cures? Some didn't think so. "We had a food fight," Farmer said. But he hadn't let himself get involved in any others.

And snow was predicted for Moscow. The news cheered him. He'd always loved a storm. "I want a blizzard!" he said.

===

Farmer had told me that playing the game of international health politics didn't come easily to him. But he was good at it, clearly, and as the days in Moscow wore on, his smiles and his vigor returned and with them, somehow, the illusion of a stylishly dressed man.

Some members of the negotiating team continued to insist that extra food for the prisoners wasn't cost-effective, but then one of the negotiators took Farmer aside and suggested that he sneak food into the budget by calling it vitamins. This worked. In the end, the World Bank team agreed that the prisoners would get about half the loan. Just now, the first installment was projected at $30 million, and the figure was bound to increase by another $100 million or so. But there might not be a loan. The Ministry of Health was bound to be displeased with their share. Still, Farmer had accomplished his main, intermediate goals, and had kept Goldfarb from executing his "Plan B."

Up in his hotel room, Farmer said, "It was a total success. I can't help but be excited. So, Alex, are you happy?"

"Yes," said Alex. "I'm always ambeevalent, though. It means I have to deal with this thirty million. Keep them from stealing it."

"They're all your friends," said Farmer. "So one of them steals for vodka and another steals for his girlfriend. Big deal."

Farmer was perched on a windowsill. Papers covered the chairs in his room. He pointed at a teetering pile of PIH stationery that an assistant had brought from Boston. "Alex, do you see the difference between your life and mine? Those are thank-you letters for twenty-five-dollar contributions to PIH."

"You do that stuff? How do you make mailing lists? Buy them?"

"Oh, come on. It's been built up over thirteen years. *You* get to write, Dear George Soros, thank you for the twelve million dollars." Farmer took up a sheaf of thank-you notes still to do and said, "I get to write to, let's see, a friend of my grandmother's, a student, a left-wing economist, an historian, a secretary in my department, an administrator in my department, a pediatrician." The recitation seemed to raise his spirits still higher. I think he was bragging, actually.

Alex's views on Farmer interested me. "Paul is so fragile," he told me privately. "He is so thin. He is like Chekhov. Sentimentality fuels him rather than otherwise. But I have never met an efficient individual who didn't claim to be sentimental or working for a higher cause. Even in business, certainly in international work."

For his part, Farmer had said of Alex, "Only a mother could love him. I do love him. I really do. And this whole thing in Russia is going to work. You know why? Because he loves me."

They seemed to have the sort of friendship that thrives on argument, and they had plenty of fodder. Take a subject like Cuba, for instance. About its health statistics, Alex said, "I think Comrade Fidel is very good at establishing discipline, so his public health must be very disciplined. I think Comrade Beria would fix the problem in Siberian prisons. Just shoot a few people."

Or take a subject like the Russian prisoners. Farmer said, "If the reason most of them are locked up is degeneracy, then how come the number of prisoners rises so much during times of great social and economic crisis or change?"

Alex saw this matter differently. At dinner one night, he remarked, "Prisoners. They are not nice people. They are epeedeemeeologically eempoortant."

"Our big split," said Farmer.

"I should take that back," Goldfarb said. "About *half* of the people should not be in jail."

"Three-quarters," said Farmer. "Come on, Alex. Those are crimes against property."

"There is twenty-five percent should be in jail for life," said Goldfarb.

"No. Ten percent," said Farmer. "You think I'm naïve."

"You are not naïve," said Goldfarb. "You see the whole situation. You just don't accept that—"

"People aren't nice."

"No! Bad people. You are not naïve. You can just disregard things which are unpleasant, and that is why you are not scientific. You disregard reality."

"But you still like me," said Farmer.

"Of course I like you!" said Goldfarb.

Farmer really did love storms, even if he rarely said so without adding that they usually afflicted the poor more than others. He had said he wished for a blizzard in Moscow. He had gotten just a snowfall. We walked back to the hotel on slippery sidewalks in the cold, cold night, Farmer with his red scarf over his nose, his glasses fogging up. We had put away three bottles of wine. I said, "You look thinner than when we started out."

"It's been a long trip," he said.

"Well, that was interesting," I said. "I like Alex."

"I'm glad. Alex is great. I was really mad at him when he first said that about prisoners, the first time I met him." He did a Russian accent: "They are bad people but epeedeemeeologically eempoortant."

I rehearsed their closing argument, Farmer's whittling down the number who he thought should be in prison. If it had gone on, I thought, he might have gotten down to one percent, or zero.

"Do you think I'm crazy?" Farmer asked.

"No. But some of those prisoners have done terrible things."

"I know," he said. "And I believe in historical accuracy."

"But you forgive everyone."

"I guess I do. Do you think that's crazy?"

"No," I said. "But I think it's a fight you can't win."

"That's all right. I'm prepared for defeat."

"But there are the small victories," I said.

"Yes! And I love them!"

My thoughts were a bit hazy, my voice, I sensed, a little slurred. I began to pose a hypothetical question, which I thought expressed great insight into his peripatetic life. "You're a great guy," I said, putting a hand on his shoulder. "But without your clinical practice—"

He interrupted. He said, "I wouldn't be anything."

Part V

O for the P

In July 2000 the Gates Foundation gave Partners In Health and a cohort of other organizations $45 million to wipe out MDR-TB in Peru, virtually everything Jim Kim had asked for. William Foege, the foundation's science adviser, the man behind the grant, liked to tell this story: Several groups all interested in the same international health problem had fought with one another for years, until he went to their leaders and said, "Gates wants to do a grant for this, but only one grant," whereupon it took about two hours for the warring factions to make peace. Jim borrowed this strategy. He included as partners some potential and former adversaries, such as WHO's tuberculosis branch. The money would be funneled through Harvard Medical School, but PIH would run the actual treatment program in Peru.

The grant would last five years. In that time, Jim figured, they'd have to treat about two thousand chronic MDR patients and cure at least 80 percent. Peru would then have control of the dread disease, and the world would have proof that countrywide control was possible and would also have the techniques and low-cost tools for accomplishing it. If all went well, that is. Partners In Health and its allies would have to convert a community health project into a national one. Inevitably there would be problems in this "scaling-up." "At times I feel like my head's going to explode," Jim told me, but he had no doubt they'd succeed.

Neither did Farmer, though he fretted some, as he did over every project, partly in this case so that Jim wouldn't get distracted but would go on fretting, too. Farmer had other, ancillary worries. When the people who had long supported PIH read about the grant—the news made the front page of *The Boston Globe*—would they think the charity didn't need their money anymore? Would some think PIH had sold its soul? In speeches to old allies and donors, Farmer began to talk about "unusual alliances." To illustrate his point, he'd show a slide of assembled photographs, in which, for instance, Fidel Castro appeared alongside the Pope, Bill Gates, and the pop singer Britney Spears. The audience would laugh, and Farmer would say, speaking of the Gates grant, "It's a wonderful thing for us, but it's very focused on our project in Peru. And we're focused on the problems of the poor. On accidents, machete wounds, burns, eclampsia. Imagine asking a foundation to support that. They'd say, 'We have a procedure and it doesn't include those things, as you'll see when you look in volume three of our grants manual.' We've had a run of luck, but it's not going to solve the problems of our sister organizations—in Chiapas, in Roxbury, in Haiti." Then he'd pause and, smiling down from the lectern at the old friends of PIH, intone, "So you are *not* dismissed."

In fact, large foundations tended to finance narrowly focused campaigns against well-publicized diseases. None was likely to be interested in simply paying the bills, year after year, for a comprehensive health care system like Zanmi Lasante. Individual donations and Tom White's dwindling fortune still were the main support for Cange, where nonetheless Farmer went on expanding his anti-AIDS campaign. Soon he had about 250 patients taking antiretrovirals there. He had grafted AIDS treatment onto Zanmi Lasante's TB program, of directly observed therapy and monthly stipends, and the early results were good—many stories of lives restored and orphanings prevented. But the waiting list of dying patients grew longer every day, and funding for antiretroviral drugs was still scarce. Though the woman he'd met in Cuba worked ardently on his behalf, UNAIDS turned down the application he'd submitted, on the grounds that his AIDS-treatment program failed to meet "sustainability criteria." That is, the drugs were too expensive for Haitians to buy for themselves in any conceivable future. Farmer got the same answer everywhere, and when he approached the drug companies, looking for donations or at least reduced prices, they suggested he go to the same agencies and foundations that had deemed his program nonsustainable because of high drug prices. He was getting by for now. Soros's foundation, which had a branch in Haiti, put up some money. Tom White made a special gift. And PIH sold its headquarters building in Cambridge, and Farmer spent most of the proceeds on drugs for treating AIDS in Cange.

Friends at Harvard Medical School had already adopted PIH and given it a second name, the Program in Infectious Disease and Social Change. (Later, not to be outdone, the Brigham would create a special division and another alias for PIH, the Division of Social Medicine and Health Inequalities.) Meanwhile, Farmer had talked the medical school into providing headquarters space for the entire growing crew, in portions of a pair of old brick buildings on Huntington Avenue, charming and warrenlike inside.

Every time I went there, I'd find that offices had moved, and soon I couldn't keep all the new names and faces straight. Just the other day, it seemed, the typical PIH-er had been a volunteer who took on chores such as finding Paul's lost luggage, then went back to analyzing epidemiological data. To meet a deadline, they'd stay all night, sleeping in shifts on a couch in the old headquarters. Now the staff included professionals in administration and information technology and grant writing, and they didn't know the PIH lingo, let alone the customs. For years Ophelia had served as the presiding spirit at headquarters, the person everyone could count on to be fair and sympathetic and, usually, temperate. Now she was trying to accommodate newcomers, trying, as Jim put it, to "normalize" the experience of working as a PIH-er: it was okay to have children, to go home some days at five o'clock, to take a vacation.

On one visit, in a new employee's office, I saw a sign taped to a wall which read, "If Paul is the model, we're golden." When you looked closely, though, you saw that the word *golden* was written on a strip of paper. Lift up the strip and you saw that the original read, "If Paul is the model, we're fucked." This was a direct quote from Jim, a characteristically emphatic phrase, which sounded harsher than it was. Jim meant it as a warning to the many young PIH-ers who imagined, as many had and many would, that the right thing to do with their lives was to imitate Paul. To Jim, attempts at imitation would put the emphasis where it didn't belong. The goal was to improve the lives of others, not oneself. "It's not about the quest for personal efficacy," as Paul himself liked to say. Besides, frank imitations would fail. What PIH-ers should take from Paul wasn't a manual for their own lives but the proofs he'd created that seemingly intractable problems could be solved. "Paul has created technical solutions to help the rest of us get to decency, a road map to decency that we can all follow without trying to imitate him," Jim told me, explaining the message on the wall. "Paul is a model *of* what should be done. He's not a model *for* how it has to be done. Let's celebrate him. Let's make sure people are inspired by him. But we can't say anybody should or could be just like him." He added, "Because if the poor have to wait for a lot of people like Paul to come along before they get good health care, they are totally fucked."

Farmer didn't disagree. I was with him one time when he was stewing over an e-mail from a student who had written that he believed in Paul's cause but didn't think he could do what Paul did. Farmer said aloud to his computer screen, "I didn't say you should do what I do. I just said these things *should* be done!" Then he framed a mild reply.

The change in PIH wasn't total. Some of the old quirkiness survived. In the old days Paul would return from a trip to Haiti, arrive at the one-room office, and the next thing Ophelia knew there would be suitcases spilling all over the floor, and everyone would be running off in various directions, doing chores for his next project. Then he'd be gone again, and she would look at Jim and say, "What just happened?" Paul still created what Ophelia called "little hurricanes." I came to the new offices once, hours after Paul had left town, and found Jim laughing, shaking his head. He had just looked in on the women who were now trying to manage Paul's schedule and travel and correspondence, and had found them in tears. Not because Paul had been cruel to them—"He's never mean," Ophelia had said, and this was true in my experience. This was a case of nervous exhaustion, a case, Jim said, of "decompressing from Paul."

The old frugality of PIH endured. The charity still used only about 5 percent of donations to administer itself, and all the rest on services to patients. Some months after they received the Gates grant, Farmer wrote an open letter to the organization. In it, he worried that PIH might be losing its way "morally." This because, among other things, some employees expected to be paid for working extra hours. He wrote, "One can never work overtime for the poor. We're only scrambling to make up for our deficiencies." Ophelia agreed in principle. She wasn't going to let PIH get bound and gagged by other institutions' rules. But she would allow some compromises, because PIH's connections to other institutions meant they could treat more patients. Their formal connection to Harvard obliged them to pay overtime to some of their lowest-salaried employees. Ophelia, who managed such matters, was following those rules. She simply didn't tell Paul.

=

About 20 people had worked at Partners In Health headquarters in Boston when I had first visited, late in 1999. Now there were 50, and another 10 in Roxbury. The numbers in Haiti had grown to about 400, and to 120 in Peru, and they were about to inherit 15 employees in Russia, because on top of everything else, PIH had expanded to Siberia.

This didn't happen by plan. It might not have happened at all if Alex Goldfarb hadn't involved himself in some mysterious relationship with the exiled Russian oligarch Boris Berezovsky. According to one published version of the story, a former KGB agent claimed he'd been ordered to assassinate Berezovsky but had tipped him off instead, allowing Berezovsky to flee Russia with his Swiss bankbooks. Later the KGB agent himself escaped, to Turkey. And then Goldfarb did Berezovsky a favor by helping the KGB agent get to London. Meanwhile, the current Russian government claimed to have a legitimate legal case against the former KGB agent, and the authorities were furious at Goldfarb. So was Soros's foundation, for putting their TB project in political jeopardy. A new director was needed anyway, because Goldfarb couldn't very well work in Russia now. He was quoted in a paper called *The Russia Journal* as saying, "Being a sane person, I would not go to Russia for a couple of weeks, at least. I'm not a fool."

After a flurry of e-mails, the foundation asked PIH to take over their project in the Siberian oblast of Tomsk. This was the site of the pilot project of pilot projects in the effort to stanch the Russian TB epidemic, the project that would show the way to controlling, in the prisons and the towns and cities, both drug-susceptible TB and MDR. "Tomsk *has* to work," Goldfarb had told me in Moscow. On that sentiment, Paul and Jim agreed. The project in Tomsk was vital. Jim was eager to add it on, even though he was already in charge of Peru and involved in the Boston projects. Paul worried. Partners In Health was stretched already. If they tried to do too much and projects faltered, there would be no end of people pointing out the failures, saying they'd shown that MDR and AIDS could not be treated in impoverished settings. But Paul agreed to take on Tomsk, provided that his role be mostly clinical, and that Jim assume the managerial chores and most of the diplomacy. Jim said he'd get to work right away, but he still hadn't gone to Russia when, about a month later, he and Paul and Ophelia went out to dinner together at a restaurant in Cambridge. I went along.

"*You* said yes to Russia," Paul told Jim, not long after we sat down. His voice had the intensity of yelling, not the full volume, but it was rising. "You fucking promised me! And you're not gonna go."

Jim protested. He had planned to travel to Tomsk this month, but it turned out he had to attend TB meetings in Bellagio, at the Rockefeller Foundation's estate on Lake Como. The meetings were crucial, Jim said.

"I don't care!" Farmer said. His neck had turned red. The veins in it stood out. "Fuck Bellagio. Bellagio, fucking Bellagio. You need to go to Moscow and Tomsk, where there's real work. You need to do some real work in Moscow. Then you can go to Bellagio and do your Harvard crap." He turned to Ophelia. "All I'm saying, Min, is that he has to go. I said, 'You won't do it, I know it, you're going to cancel, you won't go.' Now he's talking about . . . *Bellagio.* The heck with Bellagio. Lago di Como. Look, I would like to go to my *grave* never having gone to Bellagio." Paul said that Jim had gone to Moscow only once in his life, and hadn't even left the airport.

"That's not true," said Jim in a quiet voice.

"You went into town for the Bolshoi crap."

"I would have," said Jim, "but they canceled the performance."

Farmer turned to Ophelia. "They canceled the Bolshoi, Min. But he would have gone." He went on, "I'm going to go to Russia a couple of times this year, but I would like to focus on the things Jim told me I could focus on." He turned to Jim. "What were they? You tell her."

Jim smiled. "The Bolshoi and . . ."

"And dressage," said Ophelia.

Farmer didn't laugh. He said to Ophelia, "I'm asking him to limit the damage in Russia."

She said softly, "He knows that, P.J."

"Well?" said Farmer. "Force him to do it."

Jim turned to Ophelia. "He's trying to irritate me enough . . ."

"I know," she said.

The times had grown rare when all three were in the same place at the same time, but even the nostalgic talk didn't sound nostalgic tonight.

Ophelia said to Farmer, "Jim used to pick you up at the airport."

"Used to," said Paul.

"You never picked *me* up," said Jim.

"That's what he always said," Farmer announced to the table. "He said, 'You never pick *me* up.' And you were coming from Los Angeles? Sorry."

"You never did," said Jim.

"Where were you coming from?" said Paul. "You were coming from Los Angeles, or Chicago."

"Yeah, yeah," said Ophelia wearily.

"I was coming from Haiti," said Paul. "I wanted to talk to you about, what did I want to talk to you about? I talked about nothing? I always talked about Haiti."

"Anyway . . . ," said Ophelia.

"I've made my mistake," said Paul. "I'll never do it again. I'll never ask you to pick me up again."

"That's not the point," said Jim. "The point is, you never picked me up."

Ophelia told me that Paul never let himself lose his temper when it might jeopardize PIH's missions. She didn't mind that he lost it sometimes in front of her and Jim. That was safe, she thought, and also probably good for Paul's psyche. After the dinner she said to me, "You think *that* was bad? What he was doing to Jim was *nothing*. On a scale of one to ten, that was about a five." I guessed she was right. As Paul and Jim walked out the door, I saw Paul put his arm around Jim's shoulder and Jim put his arm around Paul's, and I could see they were laughing. A few weeks later, Jim flew to Siberia. I went with him.

———

It was four hours by plane from Moscow, in a Russian-made Tupo-lov 154, which had a scarred wooden toilet seat in its rest room that I figured could not be older than the plane itself. Tomsk was a city of about half a million, partially filled with Soviet constructions of steel and glass and cement block, and also with old wooden houses heaved into lopsidedness by many long winters, houses covered with fantastically ornate window casings and cornices. The city had several huge public buildings, classically porticoed. Tomsk's university was Siberia's oldest. The city had a reputable medical school and factories that made lightbulbs and matches. It had electrified trolley cars, and five competing Internet providers. But Tomsk Air had gone bankrupt, and the airport, formerly the Airport of the Workers, received not the pre-vious forty-seven flights daily but only a handful. And the water, be-cause of incipient flooding, wasn't safe to drink when we got there. Tomsk was a place where the war monuments were well-tended, and residential backyards and front yards were full of junk, poking out of the snow. We stayed in a hotel with overheated rooms and sloping floors. I had a strange dream the first night there, of a landscape full of monuments in which derelict automobiles sat on top of marble pillars.

Tomsk and the huge territory around it had a severe MDR-TB problem but one that seemed likely to be brought under control, in part thanks to Alex Goldfarb's efforts. However, because of Goldfarb's other efforts on behalf of the KGB agent, rumors were swirling around everyone who worked in the TB project, rumors that they were really spies against the motherland, part of a nefarious plot in which the patients were serving as fronts. To quell local suspicions, arrangements had been made for the vice minister of justice, who was in charge of Russia's prisons, to come to Tomsk and endorse the project and PIH's new role in it, in front of TV cameras. The vice minister had agreed to do this, a Russian general told me, because of his friendship with Farmer. A banquet was planned. Farmer was supposed to attend. He got stuck in Paris, however. His latest assistant in Boston, a young woman, had made a mistake. He couldn't get his visa until the following day. So Jim had to go it alone.

The banquet took place in what seemed like a VIP safe house, a small, luxurious private hotel tucked into a corner of a vast, gray concrete apartment and shopping complex still under construction, a part of Tomsk called, for some strange reason, Paris. The event was important. DOTS-plus would have no chance of succeeding in Russia without the ardent help of the generals who ran the prisons. Nor would the project in Tomsk, if the generals didn't trust Jim, whom they'd never met before. But a stiff formality prevailed for the first two hours or so, in spite of dozens of toasts and half a dozen bottles of vodka consumed.

The vice minister and ten big-handed Russian generals and colonels in heavy olive drab uniforms sat on one side of the assembled tables. On the other side sat the foreigners and the Russian doctors now working for PIH. The division seemed unbreachable. However, Jim had spied a TV equipped for karaoke, and as the fish course was being served I heard him whisper, "I'm gonna do it." He stood, raising his shot glass. "I'm a terrible singer, but in my culture, Korean culture, if you respect someone and you have a deep affection and admiration for the people you're with, you should embarrass yourself by singing for them. So I will sing for you."

Jim belted out "My Way." The TV orchestra accompanied him, the words scrolled across the TV screen, and then the TV got stuck, and Jim went on alone, hitting a few sour notes. Everyone clapped, and then a member of MERLIN, a British international health organization also working in Tomsk, got up and sang "Summertime," and then a two-star general ordered up a Russian song from the TV, a lively tune, the generals and the vice minister, Yuri Ivanovich Kalinin, clapping out the rhythm. Then one of the generals asked one of the Soros doctors to dance, and the Tomsk civilian TB chief, a man as large as a mature black bear, danced with a young woman from MERLIN, and Jim sang "La Bamba," and another general followed with another Russian song, while images of Broadway and bathing beauties on Caribbean beaches rolled across the TV screen. And then something rather magical happened. Without warning, and without mechanical aids, Vice Minister Kalinin himself began to sing, in a deep baritone so clear it sounded trained, a lovely, slow, and mournful-sounding ballad, and all the generals and colonels joined in. The jailers of Russia together in song. I swear it was possible, given the hour, the quantity of vodka drunk, to enjoy that spectacle of comradeship without so much as a thought about what they had all been comrades in.

I don't think I merely imagined that the farewell speeches were tinged with affection. "Dear friends," one general began. "I really mean you are my friends." Bottoms up again. Another general rose. "We have gathered around this beautiful table. All the people in the world have the same emotions. We just want to do something good for this earth." He raised his glass. "That we finish this work according to the DOTS program." He pointed to the vodka bottle in front of him. "Directly observed therapy."

Outside, snowflakes lit the air. The generals drove away with a police escort, little sedans with whirling blue lights on their roofs. Jim watched them depart, his smile like the snowflakes in the dark. "The night of the singing gulagmeisters. We're not going to see that again soon."

⸗

The next morning Jim left, and Paul arrived. He stayed only one day, which he spent examining MDR patients and giving various press conferences with the vice minister. There was another banquet that night, a smaller, quieter affair in the same strange, small hotel. At one point Vice Minister Kalinin raised his glass and said, "To Alex Goldfarb. He worked very hard and was sincere."

Farmer raised his glass. "To Alexander Davidovich. May he stay out of trouble."

Halfway through the meal, a man with tousled hair who looked like a figure in one of Goya's paintings of drunks—skin flushed, eyes squinty—wandered into the room. The interpreter leaned over to Farmer and explained that this man was a local oligarch, part owner of this place and also of Siberian gas and oil fields. The oligarch, meanwhile, was weaving his way to the head of the table. He squared his shoulders and declared, "Dear guests, I would like to say a few words. Energy is the force of life. Tomsk Oblast has oil, coal." He sucked at his teeth and corrected himself. "Tomsk doesn't have any coal, and we have to use more and more of the gas. We will be able to supply the energy needs of several oblasts."

"Bravo!" cried one of the generals.

"To the energy program!" cried Farmer.

"The moral of the story is that energy is the secret to everything in life," said the drunken interloper. "Thank you very much for coming to Siberia."

"I love Siberia!" Farmer declared from down at the other end of the table.

The oligarch lurched away. For a moment, it seemed he was leaving, but he'd only gone to get a chair. He lugged it back to the table and sat down on it heavily. "I do apologize for breaking into your life."

He cleared his throat. "I have helped a lot already. I invest a lot in culture and medicine for the city."

Other conversations resumed around the man. He seemed to be talking to himself. "What's he saying?" I asked the interpreter.

"Now he's speculating about why the Russian life is so hard."

Finally, he wandered away, and soon the farewell toasts and the good-byes began, the party moving out to the lobby. Farmer was dressed in a furry Russian hat and was saying good-bye for the third time to the vice minister. "I was very upset I wasn't here yesterday, but now I see that it's all right. We are waiting for your marching orders." He was lifting a military salute to the minister when, from a side door, the oligarch of oil and gas reappeared, naked except for a towel wrapped around his waist. He headed toward the billiard room, lurching past the vice minister, who smiled and shrugged and went back to saying good-bye. Moments later the hotel manager, a buxom woman, fully dressed and in high heels and looking greatly alarmed, came running through the lobby, pursuing the oligarch. I couldn't make out what was going on, and neither could Farmer, but, smiling gleefully, he turned and watched the chase.

We flew to Paris the next day. When we were settled in the chilly cabin of the Tupolov 154—"Has it come to this? Have we reached that age?" said Farmer as we spread blankets on our laps—I asked him a technical question about TB control, reciting an opinion I'd heard. "Would that be accurate?"

"Every account is partial." He smiled over at me. "Except mine." He went on, "I have to say, Rooskies are my kind of people."

"I've heard you say that before," I remarked.

"PIH-ers accuse me of saying it about everyone. But it comes in handy in my line of work. To like people." He made up a list of types who shouldn't be doctors. "Curmudgeons, sadists . . ."

Then he began the dismount of our short stay in Tomsk. The essence was a brief discourse on drugs. Low-cost second-line antibiotics would soon be on their way to Russia, but at the moment various snafus had delayed their arrival. Other organizations, now intent on treating MDR in Russia, were still waiting for the inexpensive drugs. Farmer and Kim, by contrast, had gone to Tom White and asked for $150,000, and bought enough drugs, at high prices, to start treating a few dozen MDR patients in Tomsk right away. Why do that, why spend $150,000 now on drugs for thirty-seven patients if, by waiting a while, they could spend the same amount and buy drugs to treat a hundred? Well, Farmer said, project managers could afford to wait for low prices, but not all patients could. "It's going to take resources to stop this epidemic," he said. "And if you want to use money to buy the resources, fine. I don't care what you use. Use cowrie shells."

Soon Farmer went to sleep. He napped most of the way to the Ural Mountains, and I tried to digest what he'd said about money. It occurred to me that PIH would probably always be in some kind of financial jeopardy, because it was constitutionally impossible for Farmer and Kim to sit on resources—to wait for lower drug prices while MDR killed Russian prisoners, to save for an endowment for Zanmi Lasante while Haitian peasants died of AIDS. Their approach, especially toward money, was completely impractical, it seemed to me, and yet it appeared to be working.

━━

Farmer was traveling more than ever. To familiar sites such as Peru and Siberia (including one trip all the way from Haiti to Tomsk for a two-hour meeting, which he considered a great success) and to Paris (where he'd agreed to give a prestigious lecture series, so as to spend more time with Didi and Catherine) and to New York (where he testified on behalf of a Haitian with AIDS who was at risk of being deported). He went to dozens of American and Canadian universities and colleges, preaching his O for the P gospel, and to South Africa, where he debated a World Bank official at an international AIDS conference. (Africans must learn to curb their sexual appetites, the banker remarked, and Farmer replied, "I want to talk about other bankers, not the World Bankers, but bankers in general. My suspicion is they're not getting a lot of sex, because they spend a lot of time screwing the poor.") He went to Guatemala to see some bodies dug up. (Partners In Health had found a donor to pay for a mental health project there: the disinterment and proper reburial of Mayan Indians who had been slaughtered by the Guatemalan army and dumped in mass graves.) One time, not long after he'd taken a fall in Cange and broken both an arm and his tailbone, he flew all the way around the world, bound for Asia on TB business.

I kept in touch with him by e-mail—he wrote almost every day— and sometimes in person. Once, in the city of San Cristóbal, in Chiapas, I stood with Ophelia and watched him from a little distance as he strode down a narrow sidewalk, a thin, long-legged white man in a black suit, weaving his way past brown-faced women in colorful Indian shawls hawking trinkets. Ophelia thought he looked like the mysterious figure at the start of a Graham Greene novel. Who was that man in the rumpled suit, and where was he going in such a hurry? I wasn't sure that the real answers would have been plausible enough for the novelist's purpose. The aim of that trip was to persuade PIH's tiny Mexican outpost to expand their public health efforts in the troubled, impoverished villages of Chiapas—an effort which, if successful, would oblige Farmer and Ophelia and Jim to do more fund-raising. And the reason he was hurrying through the streets of San Cristóbal at that moment was to get back to our hotel in time for a scheduled telephone interview with a radio station in Los Angeles, which wanted his views on AIDS.

He returned to Boston, as always, for monthlong tours of service at the Brigham. I followed him on a couple of memorable cases. A migrant worker from Mexico has been shipped to Boston from a hospital in Maine, suffering from Fournier's gangrene—a malady first described in France in the nineteenth century as "lightning gangrene of the penis." The surgeons' debridement of the dead tissue has left the man's waist and groin looking like a side of butchered beef, and some on the house staff think it's time to consider hospice care. But Farmer says cheerily, "He's going to walk out of here," and about a month later the man does. A graduate student, a young man, has arrived at the Brigham very near death. Farmer is called in and at once corrects the house staff's diagnosis. It's toxic shock, he says, and adjusts the medications. Two weeks after that the young man lies in his bed, delirious with fever, shaking so hard that from the doorway to his room I can hear his teeth chatter. The tips of his fingers and toes have turned black. And as I'm staring at him, thinking he won't make it to morning, I hear Farmer saying to the parents, "The next two weeks won't be a picnic, but the worst is over. He's going to walk out of here."

In tears, the mother says, "We trust you. Thank you so much." Two weeks later the young man's father asks if he can't repay Farmer somehow. Perhaps he can buy him a car?

He's on call one evening, driving through Boston, when his cell phone rings. "Paul Farmer. Infectious Disease," he answers. I gather the caller is another doctor, asking advice on a case. Farmer murmurs, "Uh-huh. I see." Then he asks, "Can you tell me what species of monkey it was?"

Service at the Brigham was so gratifying to him that he sometimes wondered aloud if he should give it up. Every day brought interesting cases and the pleasure of working in a hospital staffed and equipped to the highest current standards in medicine, where he could order a brain biopsy and not have to raise money to pay for it. He got medically recharged during his stopovers in Boston, but they were hardly a rest. Noting that his suit now looked like something he'd found in a trash barrel, but knowing she'd never get him to a department store, Ophelia gave his assistants a tape measure. But during most of a month he never stood still long enough for them to use it, and he left town in the same clothes.

E-mail wasn't always an enlightening means of following Farmer on his travels, because he sometimes neglected to say where he was. But one knew that most of his trips began and ended in Haiti. Some of his friends and allies continued to think he should go there far less often, and spend most of his time deploying medical troops on worldwide campaigns. Howard Hiatt felt that way more and more insistently, until he visited Zanmi Lasante. It was Dr. Hiatt's first sight of the place. When he got back to Boston, he wrote, in an editorial for

The New York Times: "I have just returned from a health center in a country at the bottom of the economic heap. . . . HIV infections are controlled as effectively in an area of Haiti as in Boston, Massachusetts. More than that, medical care there is delivered with skill and caring comparable to that seen in a Boston teaching hospital." Zanmi Lasante had moved him more deeply than anything he'd ever seen before, Hiatt told me. He said that what Paul had done in Cange had to be "replicated." And he said he intended to spend whatever time he had left on earth doing all he could to see that it was.

Replicability and sustainability—in the case of Cange, these terms had the same meaning perhaps. In Jim Kim's view, Zanmi Lasante wouldn't survive without the support of some large foundation or international agency, and it wouldn't get that support unless it was seen as something like a laboratory for the world, not just as a marvelous anomaly. At times this kind of talk made Farmer testy. "It's galling," he told me in the winter of 2002. "It should be enough to humbly serve the poor." Within a few months, though, replicating Zanmi Lasante had become his main preoccupation.

Ever since the advent of effective treatments for AIDS, in the latter 1990s, there had been debate on how and where to use the antiretroviral drugs. The argument had a grand scale and great complexity, but in fundamental ways it resembled the debates about MDR treatment—most experts saying that only prevention, not treatment, was feasible in places like Haiti and sub-Saharan Africa; others, and especially groups like ACT UP, calling the failure to treat not just immoral but also foolish, since it was clear that prevention alone would not halt the growing pandemic. To Farmer, the distinction between prevention and treatment was artificial, created, he felt, as an excuse for inaction. He had long since weighed in, in speeches and books and in dozens of journal articles. Then, in August 2001, he published an article in the British medical journal *The Lancet* describing the treatment and prevention program in Cange. At once PIH began receiving requests for advice and information—at one point I counted nearly one hundred. They came from ministries of health and consultants and charities from every continent. The Harvard "Consensus Statement," an argument for worldwide treatment, which 140 of the faculty signed, cited the project in Cange. The new chief of WHO's TB division praised it in a letter to *The New York Times*. Meanwhile, the economist Jeffrey Sachs was dispersing the *Lancet* article far and wide.

Sachs had visited Zanmi Lasante himself, and he'd had much the same reaction as Howard Hiatt. Sachs wrote to me,

> Paul's work (and his concept of high-quality medical care for the poor) has had a *huge* effect. I was able to use the example of his work in many key fora around the world in the past few years, with the U.S. Congress, the WHO Commission on Macroeconomics and Health, the White House, the U.S. Treasury, United Nations Secretary General Kofi Annan, etc. When I worked with the Secretary General to help launch the Global Fund to Fight AIDS, Tuberculosis and Malaria, Paul's work was a key example.

"It's embarrassing that piddly little projects like ours should serve as exemplars," Farmer told me. "It's only because other people haven't been doing their jobs." It did seem like a case of gross disproportion in cause and effect. In the world, about 40 million people were infected with HIV, and a program that was treating only hundreds of those in rural Haiti had somehow acquired great weight. But Zanmi Lasante's program was in fact unique, at least at the time of Farmer's *Lancet* article. Other small AIDS-treatment and -prevention programs were under way in poor countries, but Zanmi Lasante's was the only one in an impoverished rural area that chose its patients solely on medical grounds and not on their ability to pay, the only one that provided expert care and treatment for free.

The Global Fund, which Sachs helped to create, was a brand-new institution, financed by governments and foundations. The hope was to raise many billions of dollars annually to fight the world's three great pandemics. By the spring of 2002, it had collected pledges for only a fraction of the goal. Nevertheless, the fund had begun receiving applications for grants and approved, among others, Haiti's application, which PIH had helped to write. According to the plan, Zanmi Lasante would direct a thorough AIDS-treatment and -prevention program through most of the central plateau. The project would, it was hoped, serve as a model for similar projects in Haiti's eight other departments and in other very poor countries.

Every part of the task looked daunting, and politics promised to make the job both harder and more pressing. When President Aristide's government had been restored in 1994, a host of nations and international development banks had pledged their help in rebuilding Haiti. But contributions were already dwindling by the time of Aristide's reelection, in late 2000. Now the United States was leading a concerted effort to block aid to Haiti's government—not just American aid but also grants and loans from other sources, including loans from an international agency that would have financed an increase in the supplies of potable water and improvements in roads, education, and the public health system. The stated reasons for this policy were various and changeable. The real reasons probably included long-standing institutional fear and distrust of Aristide, a hope that Haitians might blame him for the country's continuing decline, and general weariness with Haiti's problems. Farmer wrote to me, about the blocked loans: "I think, sometimes, that I'm going nuts, and that perhaps there *is* something good about blocking clean water for those who have none, making sure that illiterate children remain so, and preventing the resuscitation of the public health sector in the country most in need of it." He added, "Lunacy is what it is."

In Cange at least, the effects of dwindling aid seemed plain. By 2002 the public clinics out in the central plateau had all but shut down for lack of cash. Impoverished peasant families had nowhere to go but Cange. They were flocking to Zanmi Lasante in overwhelming numbers, four times as many as just two years before. Patients filled every hospital bed at the complex, and every reclining chair, and every space on the floors. In effect, the people of the central plateau were begging Zanmi Lasante to do the same thing as the Global Fund asked.

Just to enact one part of the plan, just to extend Zanmi Lasante's program for preventing transmission of HIV from mothers to babies, looked as difficult as the nationwide MDR project in Peru, and that project ranked among the most complex health interventions ever undertaken in a poor country. Only 20 percent of women in rural Haiti received any medical care. An estimated 5 percent had HIV. To find them, Farmer's team, a group of PIH and Zanmi Lasante doctors and health workers and Haitian government employees, would have to undertake AIDS education among about half a million peasants who were scattered throughout a mountainous region of about four hundred square miles. They'd have to establish labs and testing centers in a place where the principal roads were nearly impassable even in good weather. ("As for transportation," Farmer wrote to PIH-ers, "we believe it's gonna be donkey & bike & motorcycle & jeep.") They'd have to train lab technicians to run those centers, in places that had only intermittent electricity or none, and hire and train many additional community health workers to deliver prophylactic drugs twice a day for nine months to each infected pregnant woman and for a week to each newborn baby. Because breast milk can transmit the virus, each mother would have to be provided with infant formula for at least nine months, and because the formula would have to be mixed with local water, Farmer's team would have to clean up the water supplies in dozens of places.

The Global Fund money—$14 million for the central plateau, paid out over five years—would go mainly for anti-HIV drugs and for hiring Haitian health workers and for fixing up the few public clinics that already existed in the region. But treating and preventing HIV would also mean treating and preventing tuberculosis. And when they set up clinics to treat those two diseases, people would come to them with other ailments, with broken legs and machete wounds, with typhoid and bacterial meningitis. A PIH project couldn't refuse to treat people who didn't have the right diseases. So they'd have to spread facsimiles of the medical complex in Cange throughout the vast, mountainous, famished Département du Centre, and if they were lucky and frugal, $14 million would get them started.

But Farmer was elated. When he got word about the Global Fund money, he wrote to me, "I feel like weeping. The Haitians so deserve this." He wrote that he would study his schedule and cancel whatever he could so as to spend more time in Haiti. A few weeks later he was in Tomsk, visiting patients and checking out the program there. Not long after that, he was in Barcelona, addressing the annual international conference on AIDS.

Once, arriving in Boston, exhausted after another of his light months for travel, Farmer told Ophelia that he heard two sets of voices. At one ear he heard friends and allies saying he should concentrate on the big issues of world health and, at the other ear, the groans of his Haitian patients: the voice of the world saying, "This meeting's important," and the voice of Haiti saying, "My child is dying." Once in a while, cramped in an airplane seat, he had talked to me about retiring to Cange, about wanting to stay put there and be "just a country doctor." I didn't fully believe him. For as long as he could manage the travel, I thought, he'd be leaving Haiti for places like Tomsk and Lima, to doctor individual patients and to do his part fighting plagues and inequities in health, practicing his own combination of wholesale and retail medicine. But he'd always return to Cange. It seemed to me that he didn't have a plan for his life so much as he had a pattern. He was like a compass, with one leg swinging around the globe and the other planted in Haiti.

CHAPTER 25

The transit between Cange and Boston used to jar Farmer back when he was a young medical student. He'd leave peasant huts full of malnourished babies and, arriving in Miami Airport, overhear well-dressed people talk about their efforts to lose weight. The trip was unsettling in either direction. One day he'd be inside the teaching hospitals of Boston, receiving instruction in the highest current standards of medical care, and the next morning he'd be climbing out of a tap-tap, his face gray with dust, into the squatter settlement in the parched high ground above the dam, where there was no medicine, let alone standards of care. In time he learned to make the transition more calmly. "After a while I realized I could do just as good a job treating my patients without getting angry," he told me. By then, I think, he was transmuting anger into something that felt better, a dream of ending the disparities, at least the medical ones, that separated Boston and Cange.

The dream seemed impossible, of course, but he still held to it. "I don't mean we should do bone-marrow transplants in Cange, but proven therapies," he'd say in lectures. "Equity is the only acceptable goal." He had made progress. Zanmi Lasante now had decent facilities, including a good operating room, always sparkling clean. But it still lacked a lot of high-tech equipment. There was no blood bank, no CT scanner. Farmer intended to fix those deficiencies and more, someday. In the meantime, on occasion, when he couldn't bring Boston medicine to Cange, he'd bring a patient from Cange to Boston.

In early 2000, PIH had flown a young man named Wilnot to the Brigham. He had a rare congenital heart defect, which a team of surgeons fixed, waiving their fees. Several months later, near the beginning of August, a woman from the city of Hinche, eschewing the dreadful public hospital there—floors of rotting wood, an open sewer out back, no medicine without cash—brought her son by tap-tap over the road to Zanmi Lasante. The boy's name was John. Like their deaths, the births of most Haitian peasants go unrecorded, so John's exact age was uncertain. He was probably eleven or twelve. He and his mother were all that remained of their immediate family. John's father and his three siblings had all died during the past few years, apparently of various ailments. When asked what he thought those had been, Farmer adapted a mordant line from Graham Greene's *The Comedians*. "Haiti," he said. "They died of Haiti." John's mother called her life "a series of catastrophes." Though far from unprecedented, the family history lent John's case a special urgency. The clinical facts made it singular.

John had swellings in his neck, which at first glance resembled scrofula—cervical lymphadenitis, TB in the lymph nodes of the neck, fairly common in Haiti. But with scrofula the nodes feel squishy. John's felt hard to Farmer's touch. And the proportion of white cells in his blood was much higher than usually seen in extrapulmonary TB. Farmer suspected some sort of cancer.

A diagnosis that would take a few hours in Boston can take weeks when made between Haiti and Boston. Serena Koenig, a Brigham doctor in her early thirties, had arranged for Wilnot's operation and the fund-raisers that had paid for his travel and hospital stay. Now Serena found an oncologist at Massachusetts General Hospital who agreed to make the diagnosis for free. Of course, the oncologist needed a sample of tissue from John. Obtaining the tissue involved a tricky surgical procedure, one that Farmer didn't feel he should perform himself, if he had a choice. He sent word to a Haitian surgeon in Mirebalais, one he knew to be competent. The surgeon agreed to come to Cange, for several thousand dollars, a very large fee in Haiti. It was raining in the central plateau, and fetching the surgeon meant braving the mud and swollen streams between Mirebalais and Cange. The trip took twelve hours. The biopsy lasted until dawn. Farmer was scheduled to fly to Boston that morning. He brought John's blood and tissue samples with him, and Serena took them to Mass General in a plastic shopping bag. Zanmi Lasante didn't have the equipment to preserve the specimens in frozen sections, so they'd been placed in formaldehyde. This meant that the diagnosis itself took four days instead of just one.

The news was bad. John had nasopharyngeal carcinoma, a very rare cancer, constituting less than 1 percent of all childhood malignancies. If caught early, however, 60 to 70 percent could be cured.

At first Farmer thought they could treat John in Haiti, adminstering the chemotherapy in Cange. He got Serena to obtain the regimen from her contacts at Mass General. She was about to start buying the drugs—cisplatin, methotrexate, leucovorin—when an oncologist friend in Boston told her, "Serena, if you want to kill this child, there are less painful ways to do it." In fact, only a handful of hospitals in the United States had the right equipment and experience to deal properly with John's illness. So Serena and Farmer agreed they'd try to bring the boy to Boston. Farmer was very busy, of course, and had to follow a lot of the case from a distance. Serena did almost all the work. The hospital bill for John would come to something like $100,000. Serena begged and cajoled nonstop for three weeks. Finally, the authorities at Mass General agreed to take the case for free.

But by now a month had passed since John's mother had brought him to Cange. Serena still had to put together a pile of documents, for Mass General and for the American consulate in Haiti so that she could get a visa for John. She didn't even know John's parents' first names. There was no more time to lose, so Serena made up names— Jean Paul and Yolande. Serena didn't speak Creole, and she figured that since John had never traveled beyond the central plateau he was bound to be scared, flying to America without his mother. She knew a Haitian American, a resident in internal medicine and pediatrics at Mass General and the Brigham, named Carole Smarth. Carole had spent parts of her childhood in Haiti, she spoke Creole fluently, and she was a friend of PIH—she'd worked for a few weeks at Zanmi Lasante. She agreed to go to Cange with Serena and help fetch John to Boston.

Serena called Farmer, who was traveling. She was afraid John might have grown much sicker in the past month and she asked Farmer what circumstances would keep them from bringing John to Mass General.

"No circumstances," Farmer said. "It's his only chance."

"What will I say if I'm asked why we're doing this?"

"That his mother brought him to us," said Farmer. "And we're doing everything we can to help him."

$=$

Serena's first sight of Haiti had horrified her. Zanmi Lasante had moved her. The whole experience of bringing Wilnot to Boston had changed her life, she felt. She was still employed by the Brigham and Harvard Medical School, but now spent most of her free time working for Paul and Jim.

PIH-ers weren't all alike, of course, but many had impressive academic credentials, many were religious, the majority were female, and a lot of those were, as Ophelia said, "rather good-looking." The full description fit both Serena and Carole. As I hurried along with these two young doctors through Logan Airport, I noticed a lot of people glancing our way.

Serena had brought two suitcases, one full of stuffed animals and toys for the pediatric ward in Cange. Carole had brought a gigantic bag, a bag of Haitian-returning-from-the-United-States proportions. It was filled with medicines she thought they might need to get John safely through the trip. Carole also carried a plastic bag filled with water. Two shebunkins were finning around inside, goldfish for Farmer's new fish pond at his house in Cange. He'd asked that some be brought, if it wasn't too much trouble.

He wouldn't be there when we arrived. He had to go to Europe for a scientific meeting; the head of Soros's foundation had asked him to go, and he'd felt he couldn't refuse. Right now he was in a German castle, of all places. But his young colleagues were certifiably first-rate doctors from two of the world's best teaching hospitals, and it looked to me as though they'd thought of everything. Serena had been too busy with arrangements to sleep last night. Now she ran through the whole list of what she'd done and was still reciting it when we got on the plane.

The plan was to get John a visa on arriving in Port-au-Prince, drive on to Cange, and bring him back to Boston the next day—in first class, with Carole sitting beside him. Farmer, always saving money so there would be more money to spend, had insisted by e-mail that they not buy first-class tickets but use some of his own vast store of frequent-flyer miles.

The first part of the plan unwound smoothly, largely because of Ti Fifi, one of Farmer's best and oldest Haitian friends, the person whom, above all, he could count on to get a thing done in Haiti. The Haitian Godfather, Farmer called her. Ti Fifi was small and quiet, usually smiling. When she met us at the airport, she said she'd managed to get John a Haitian passport. First, she'd had to manufacture a birth certificate. Serena said, "If you get him another one, could you make his mother's name Yolande?"

Everyone laughed. I myself felt a lack of reserve that should have made me nervous. I felt as if I were slipping into a holiday mood, embarked on another vicarious moral adventure, which looked as though it would be painless. The American consulate granted the visa at once. Then, late in the afternoon, we headed north toward Cange, in the Zanmi Lasante truck.

Nearly a year ago I'd seen a sign at the foot of Morne Kabrit where the paving gave out, a sign that announced the imminent rehabilitation of National Highway 3. Now rust from the fastenings dripped down the face of the sign, but it was still in better shape than the road. Some rocks had been moved around at the foot of the mountain, but not an inch of the track had been smoothed or paved, and all the earthmoving equipment was gone, except for one machine parked about a third of the way up the slope, on its way to becoming a relic.

"What happened?" I asked Ti Fifi.

She shrugged. She'd heard that the European and South American contractors had either wasted all the money or stolen it.

A battered old truck had turned over on the road up the mountain, blocking the way. There was a traffic jam of tap-taps and *camions,* the truck's carcass at the center and a crowd milling around it. After a lot of arguing and failed attempts, in which a few people nearly got crushed, the crowd rolled the truck off to one side of the road. All that took a while. It was after dark when we turned in at Zanmi Lasante's gate and I felt again the relief of smooth pavement, by now a familiar pleasure, a secure feeling, which this time didn't last. Serena and Carole went right up to the Children's Pavilion. The place felt different from the last time I'd been there. The hospital didn't look quite as clean or the walls as white, and the air inside seemed hotter, the flies thicker. But I don't think anything had changed in fact. I think it was just that Farmer wasn't there. The hospital seemed less reliable without him. And the sight of John in his bed shocked me.

In photographs taken a month before, he had looked merely sick. Now his legs and arms were emaciated. You could see all the bones in them, and his knee and elbow joints looked outsize, with the flesh shrunk away. He'd been given a tracheotomy. A round peg to accommodate a feeding tube was fixed in the front of his neck, on either side of which bulb-shaped lumps of flesh stood out. The swellings forced his tongue from his mouth. He was shifting around, clearly trying to find a way to take the pressure off his neck. He made a gurgling sound—secretions clogging his airways. A nurse suctioned them out with an electrical device. On top of everything else, he was running a fever.

I couldn't look at him again right away. I glanced around the room instead, and found myself staring at a baby with kwashiorkor in the crib near the stairs. Her eyes looked immense, like the eyes of a frightened woodland creature. I looked at John's mother, a dark-skinned, very thin woman. She sat on the side of the bed, staring at nothing, it seemed, no expression at all on her face. I looked at Serena and saw that she, too, was looking away—gazing at the wall above John's bed, her lips pursed. She was silent for a long moment, which seemed to stretch into minutes. Then she thrust her hands through her hair and said, "Okay, we need to know why he has a fever, what meds he's on." She started leafing through John's records, and Carole went to John's bedside.

The boy was gesturing at Carole's black purse. He wanted to see what was in it. Carole opened it and held it toward him. He poked his fingers around inside, then waved dismissively at it, as if to say, Nothing interesting in there.

Carole leaned over him and spoke softly in Creole. *"Pa pè"*—"Don't be afraid," she said, and tears began to roll down John's cheeks, pearly in the dim light of the Children's Pavilion.

The two doctors and Ti Fifi moved away from the bed to confer. "The most reassuring thing to me right now is he's totally a kid," said Carole. She went on, "His spleen and liver are not enlarged. The only thing is his congestion."

"I think the congestion will be better with him sitting up," Serena said. She was thinking about trying to get him on the plane tomorrow. Maybe she could cover his neck with a blanket. The image didn't work, though. "I don't think we can take him on a commercial airline. I don't think they'd let him on board. So why don't we just figure out how we take him on another plane? Carole, do we or do we not take him tomorrow on a commercial plane?"

"The one thing that's going to kill him are these secretions," said Carole. "I think it would be irresponsible, as a physician, to take him. Without suction. On a plane."

Serena went over the situation. The chief pediatric oncologist at Mass General had told her that John had a reasonable chance if the cancer had not metastasized into his bones, and there was no way of telling, here in Cange, if that had happened. "He has to have his fighting chance," Serena said.

Ti Fifi said, "Maybe we can get a helicopter to Port-au-Prince and then a medevac flight." She looked thoughtful. "I don't know what a medevac flight will cost."

"Maybe twenty thousand dollars," said Carole.

"Let's just pay it," said Serena. "Now I'm like, big deal, what's twenty thousand? What if he died on the plane? I can see the story. Harvard doctors from PIH totally irresponsible. Jim would kill me. I shouldn't have left this little boy here a month ago. I feel very responsible. Next time I'll be quicker."

"We didn't even have a diagnosis a month ago," said Carole.

"I'm just bummed because I should have brought him back a month ago," said Serena. "We dicked around waiting for a diagnosis."

Carole looked down. The plastic bag with Farmer's new shebunkins was sitting on the floor. "Shit! I brought them all this way, they're not going to die now."

They took a break and walked across the *gwo wout la* with flashlights to Farmer's *ti kay* and turned on the lights to his fish pond. Carole looked down into the plastic bag and said, "That's Jean Claude and Yolande. I'll miss you, too, kids, but you gotta go ahead and make some friends." She dumped them in the pond, and we bent over and watched the fish swim off among the others.

———

At dawn Serena and Ti Fifi headed back to Port-au-Prince, to look for a medevac and a helicopter. It was a long day.

When the truck reached the paved road at the foot of Morne Kabrit, Alix, Zanmi Lasante's driver, accelerated to seventy miles an hour and went into the city scattering chickens and dwarf goats. He pulled out into oncoming traffic to pass *camions* and tap-taps, making a third lane on the road, which had only two, and sometimes making a fourth as he pulled out to pass vehicles that had themselves pulled out to pass. Carole had said there was a special beep that drivers made on their horns in Port-au-Prince to announce, "I'm coming around this corner in the wrong lane," and the saying in her girlhood was that if you made that beep and then heard another like it coming from the other direction, you prayed you would die in the collision so as not to be sent to the Central Hospital.

I told myself that, if I were a Haitian, I'd compete wildly to get a leg up on anything I could, and probably be an anarchic driver, too. And then I thought that here were Serena and Ti Fifi trying to save a boy's life, while Alix, sweetly smiling at the wheel, was putting dozens of other lives in jeopardy, just now those of two boys sharing a bicycle, the truck's side mirror nearly brushing their shoulders. When we got stuck in the traffic near the airport, I felt relieved, for a while.

We were in and out of traffic jams all day, traveling to Ti Fifi's family's house in the city, where there was a computer hooked up to the Internet, then to the airport, then to the office of a friend of Ti Fifi's who had a fax machine, then back to the airport, then back to her place. There was lots of time to see the sights by the sides of the city roads. The brightly painted wooden booths selling lottery tickets, the proprietors' hopes preying on hope—"Bank Lotto, New York." The rubble by the sides of the streets—old tires, trash, ragged chunks of concrete, skeletons of trucks and cars stripped as clean as bones in a desert. Men sitting with shotguns on their knees outside every gas station. Dying men and women begging. People on crutches, people with the stumps of their legs inserted in what looked like ice cream containers. Up ahead in traffic, I saw a *camion* with a legend painted on its rear window which seemed to sum up Serena and Ti Fifi's problem for today. "Oh Morne Kabrit!" it read.

A medevac flight from Port-au-Prince to Boston was fairly easy to arrange. It entailed only several phone calls and one traffic jam. But the price was $18,540. Serena was ready to pay it and raise the money later, but Ti Fifi wanted Farmer's approval. Serena had sent him this e-mail: "John's condition is growing more tenuous. He is curious, sweet as can be, interactive with us and they would not have let him on the plane. And yet weak weak weak and I fear would not survive the trip to the airport and they would not have let him on the plane. Polo, I know this sounds crazy but he still has his fighting chance. This could still be a localized tumor with abscess tipping him over and increased mass size. I will take responsibility to pay for this flight. We are proceeding with plan while we wait to hear from you."

But Farmer seemed worried about the expense, and perhaps the precedent, of a medevac flight. He'd written back, "Serena, honey, please consider other possibilities."

This message left Ti Fifi looking worried, which was unusual. Sitting by her computer, she said, "Usually Paul would say, 'I trust you. Go ahead.' He would never say don't do it. But if he wanted us to do it, he would say so."

"So in the context of Polo, this is a no," said Serena.

"It's close," said Ti Fifi. "There's other consequences to this. What are we going to do if another kid like this comes to us? It's not a one-time thing. We're not going to close the hospital after this. It's really tricky. The staff will be asking why did they spend this money. Paul's worried about it."

"I'm looking at only one child," Serena said.

"That's the thing," said Ti Fifi. "There are so many kids waiting for heart surgery, and the staff is asking for more money. A medevac flight is not something you do in Haiti." Softly, as if to herself, she added, "I am sure that people will say, If your child is sick go to Cange and they will fly him to Boston. In the central plateau, this is going to be an event."

"I have an idea!" said Serena. "Just have me pay for it, and tell everyone in Cange that I did." She added, "The fact that he has free care at the other end makes it excruciating."

"We should get all the arrangements and the cost, and ask Paul," said Ti Fifi. "Because I know this guy."

Serena seemed on the verge of tears. Ti Fifi got up and hugged her. Ti Fifi, whose head barely reached the level of Serena's shoulders, reaching up, Serena bending her knees to receive the hug. Ti Fifi laughed softly, saying, "More and more patients. Every day something. A crisis. Like John. This is nothing. Every day, every minute you have cases like this. Someone's sick, someone's in danger."

Then Ti Fifi got on the computer and wrote Farmer, "You have to say yes or no."

I imagined him receiving this message, restive in a Bavarian castle. His reply came fairly quickly. He wrote, of the cost of the medevac,

"Well, it could be worse." Also: "I'll be there within twenty-four hours, but would not try to second-guess all of you there. Getting him on a plane is the only way to save his life, so I'm for it." He closed, "In any case, his hope is in leaving Haiti, by one way or another—like many other Haitians, alas."

But there was still the matter of getting John down Highway 3 to Port-au-Prince. "He will die on the road," one of Zanmi Lasante's Haitian doctors had said last night. This seemed far from unlikely to me. Ti Fifi had searched through the airport for someone with a helicopter, but there appeared to be none in Haiti, at least none available to her—and she was very well-connected. Perhaps a small plane would do—but no landing strip existed anywhere near Cange. So John would have to be taken down the road, over its boulders and giant potholes, across the streams. Ti Fifi didn't like the prospect. "I'm not giving up," she said to Serena. "But what is best for John?"

"He will be in his mother's lap in the truck," said Serena. "Ti Fifi, I know he looks very weak, but I think it's criminal not to try."

"Okay," said Ti Fifi.

"The reason I feel so strongly about it is I talked to Paul about this."

"Paul is not here," said Ti Fifi. She sighed, then smiled. "There's no point arguing. It's the same, you know, circle."

"If only we'd brought manual suction," said Serena. This now looked like the insuperable problem. Without a suctioning device, John might well asphyxiate on the trip to Port-au-Prince, and the only suctioning devices in Cange were electrical. None would work in the truck.

Ti Fifi wondered if they could hire an ambulance with its own device. She worked her contacts and found a publicly owned ambulance that would have done the job for free, if it hadn't been broken down and in the shop. Ti Fifi shook her head and smiled at this news. "Only God, only God can help us," she said. Then she got on the phone again and located a private ambulance company.

It was on John Brown Avenue, an outfit called Sam's Service Ambulance. The company owned one vehicle. It was shiny but old—a

Kennedy, a recycled American model from around the 1970s, and it didn't have four-wheel drive.

Nevertheless, Ralph, the proprietor, was willing to try the road to Cange. He was a fit-looking, muscular fellow. He'd served in the U.S. Army for ten years and had come back to Haiti to build a little business—hoping, he said, to do his part to help his native country. But while Haiti had plenty of need for ambulances, there weren't many people who could pay for one, and he'd grown discouraged. Why not, he seemed to feel, give this job a try?

He and four of his men got dressed for the journey. They put on T-shirts that read "Sam's Service Ambulance" and white hard hats, and climbed into their vehicle. Then they turned on their siren and led the way out of Port-au-Prince at high speed, calling back, "Follow us!" through the loudspeaker mounted on their roof.

The ambulance broke down for the first time about halfway up Morne Kabrit. It was dark and pouring rain by then. Sitting in the Zanmi Lasante truck, parked on the edge of the cliff, we watched one of Ralph's men pour quart after quart of oil into the ambulance's engine. The headlights of both vehicles angled sharply upward. I noticed the rainwater. It was running with the volume of a small brook down the so-called road, a dry riverbed no more, and I wondered what would happen if the rain didn't stop. And what about the *zenglendo,* the bandits who were said to prey on broken-down travelers? Ti Fifi was a very calm person, and even she had said she didn't like to be out on the *gwo wout la* after dark, because of the *zenglendo.* But Farmer had said that Haitians don't like being out in the rain, and maybe this generalization applied to *zenglendo,* too.

We sat inside the truck waiting for about half an hour. No ambulance meant no suction device. For the lack of a simple manually operated tool, all the work would be spoiled and the boy's life forfeit. I was immersed in these thoughts when Serena said, "Well, guys, we did it. He's flying out tomorrow."

I said, "Serena, that isn't clear yet."

"But you gotta rejoice a little along the way," she said. Then she started in on worries that seemed remarkably premature. "We have to have the ambulance get to Port-au-Prince right when the plane arrives tomorrow. So that John gets to Mass General before five P.M. if possible, because . . ."

I muttered, I'm ashamed to say, that Sam's Service Ambulance wasn't going to make it up Morne Kabrit, never mind to Cange, and Serena began to cry. Then, just as I'd begun to apologize, Ti Fifi's cell phone rang. It was Ralph calling from a few yards away.

"They're still going to try?" Serena asked.

"I guess so," said Ti Fifi.

"Oh, I love them!" said Serena.

Ti Fifi chuckled. "God is good."

But about two-thirds of the way to the summit, the ambulance stopped again. In the stage set that our headlights made, you could see steam pouring out from under the hood. A couple of Ralph's men came outside in their hard hats and ponchos and rolled a large rock behind one of the ambulance's wheels. Ti Fifi's cell phone rang again.

"They have tried," Ti Fifi said to Serena. "But now they are low on oil again, and they don't have any more."

"But maybe they'll loan us their suction," said Serena.

"If they will, we will have to pay them something," said Ti Fifi.

"Pay them *lots,*" said Serena.

After a little palaver, Ralph said, "No problem." Serena was cheerful again. She and Ti Fifi got out and climbed into the back of the ambulance to watch the men work. Inside the Zanmi Lasante truck, Patrice, one of the hospital workers, shook his head. "I think Serena, she never gives up."

A female version of Farmer in this respect, I thought. But I didn't see what good it would do to transfer the suction device. It was electrical. It would take better mechanics than these guys to hook it up to Zanmi Lasante's truck, in the middle of the night, during a rainstorm on the slopes of Morne Kabrit.

Hours—it seemed like hours—went by. The rain had let up. I stood outside and listened to Ralph and his men at work. There was a lot of banging and scraping. It sounded as if they were tearing the whole ambulance apart. I poked my head inside the back door and heard Ralph say to Ti Fifi, "You should have me run transportation for your hospital, and I'm tellin' you, *no* problems."

I thought, Yeah, sure, as you mangle your broken-down ambulance. It is so easy, at least for me, to mistake a person's material resources for his interior ones.

I stood at the edge of the cliff and gazed at the lights of Port-au-Prince far below. More time went by, and then I saw Serena's hand appear out of the back of the ambulance with the thumb turned upward, and moments later Ralph was carrying the suction device to the truck. He had mounted it on a board and wired it to a plug that would fit the socket of the truck's cigarette lighter. He leaned into the cab, inserted the plug, and the machine began whirring. Serena clapped her hands.

Then Ti Fifi said we should go back to Port-au-Prince for the night and get another truck, because there would be no room for Serena and me and Patrice inside this one tomorrow, and Serena said, "No. We can't do that. It would mean another day's delay." She and I would ride to the airport tomorrow in the open bed of the truck. "That's what Paul would say. Get your ass in the back."

The streams that cross Highway 3 were swollen. They looked like rapids in the headlights, and Alix actually paused at the first one, then plunged the truck in. For a moment our lights were shining through water, and then we were across. Later Serena would tell me that she had been very frightened. "What if I die?" she said she had thought, when the headlights went underwater. "I can't die," she had answered herself. "I have so much life left." And then, as the truck had struggled up onto dry land, shuddering like a beast shaking off water, she'd said to herself, "Okay, remember that. If it's *your* life, it's always the most important thing."

—

The party made an early start for Port-au-Prince the next morning. As usual, there was a crowd of patients in the courtyard. They watched solemnly as Dr. Hugo Jerome carried John in his arms out to the truck. He kissed the boy, then placed him in the backseat beside his mother and Carole. Dr. J, as I called him, was one doctor who, I believed, would never leave Cange for a better posting—one time in my presence he'd raised a glass of Haitian rum and said to Farmer, "You are the best Haitian I know."

Alix rose to the occasion. He drove very slowly over the craters of Highway 3, and the long stretches of lumpy, fissured bedrock, and the steep inclines where the dirt track was just piles of boulders. Inside the truck Carole and John's mother ministered to the boy. He suffered, every bump a sharp pain. "Imagine your worst sore throat times a thousand," Carole said. But the suction device never quit, and John arrived safely at the airport, and safely in Boston, perhaps the first Haitian peasant ever to have traveled in a Learjet. At Logan an ambulance came onto the tarmac and picked us all up. I rode in front with the driver. He told me, "It's gonna get real rough."

"How so?"

"The roads. There's a lot of bad road between here and Mass General."

This should have been comic, but I couldn't begin to explain that to the driver, and for some reason I couldn't name, this made me sad.

The little jet had landed once, in Wilmington, North Carolina, so we could all clear customs. The agent had asked Serena the perfunctory question, "Did you bring anything back from Haiti?" Then the agent had added, "Not that you'd get anything there anyhow, except disease."

Back in the plane, Serena had said, "I wanted to slug her right in the nose. But I'm a total pacifist."

In Wilmington, Serena had put on a dress. Her other clothes had been soiled with dust from the *gwo wout la*. "I can't go into Mass General looking like this," she had said. She was worried enough as it was, about what the nurses and doctors there would say when they saw John. It was a prescient worry.

The team at the pediatric intensive care unit was quick and deft, and had John in bed in an instant, but Serena overheard one of the doctors on duty say over the phone to her boss, "He's all neck and bones!" And so when Farmer called, from Haiti, Serena said, "Hey, we did the *right* thing." Farmer was agreeing emphatically, I could tell, and Serena said again, "So, Polo, we did the right thing, I have no doubt we did the right thing."

In a little while Serena and I went to a room nearby to eat the hospital supper. An intern, a young woman, joined us. She looked very young, indeed almost adolescent, and she was just out of medical school, whereas Serena was an attending physician at the Brigham. But the intern was clearly too upset to care about protocol. Hadn't they been feeding this child in Haiti? she asked. "I'm shocked," she said. She added, as if lecturing a student, "Dying from chemotherapy is terrible, you know."

Serena pursed her lips. She had begun to try to explain—one had to understand what Haiti was like and how hard it was to get someone back from there, and of course John was malnourished, but Paul Farmer, who was a famous doctor, had ordered that John be fed aggressively and had even arranged for a feeding tube, which was something rarely done in Haiti, but even the head pediatric oncologist at Mass General had said that no amount of nourishment would fatten up a child afflicted with this kind of cancer, and John still had his fighting chance—when a small, trim, middle-aged man in a black suit walked into the room. Dr. Alan Ezekowitz, the head of pediatrics. I wondered if he could possibly have overheard the intern lecturing Serena because the first thing he said, in a loud, brassy voice, smiling at Serena, was, "Well, this boy is a challenge. But I've cured sicker kids."

Serena laughed nervously. She said, "Well, now he's in Man's Greatest Hospital." That was what Mass General people called the place, playing on its initials, MGH.

Dr. Ezekowitz chuckled. "As soon as we start to believe that, we won't be." He turned to the young intern. "Isn't that right? We can always do better, can't we."

The intern bowed her head. "Yes, Dr. Ezekowitz."

=

The next afternoon Serena called me and said that a formidable phalanx of radiologists, pediatricians, and cancer doctors had just spent an
hour studying John's X rays and bone scans and CT scans. Then,
weeping over the phone, she said, as if all in one breath: "It's everywhere. It's in his mouth, it grows into the vertebral bodies. The poor
kid has been in horrible pain. It started at the nasal area, just one solid
tumor, growing back into the spinal column, the roof of the mouth.
You can't radiate four vertebral bodies. So he's gonna die. He's getting
excellent care, but there's still a bit of why did you bring him? Why?
Because, A, he's a human being, and B, because I didn't know he
couldn't be treated, and C, why shouldn't he have a comfortable way
to die, why shouldn't his mother have a private room without flies on
her face to grieve in? Can we not have him in a place where people are
trained in palliation? Isn't palliative care important? And a place where
his mother can grieve in private instead of an open ward with flies all
over her face?"

John did get first-rate care, of course, and all the right drugs at the
right doses so that he was never in apparent pain again. Serena and
Carole spent most of the next two weeks in his room, taking turns
sleeping there on a cot. John's favorite toy was a broken child's tape
recorder which had a play phone attached. He'd pick it up and speak
into it.

"Who are you talking to?" Carole asked him in Creole.

"My mother."

"What are you telling her?"

"Vini, vini." "Come quick." He motioned for Carole to say the
same words over the phone, and she did, and he was satisfied.

His mother arrived within several days, along with Ti Fifi, who had
made the arrangements. Farmer spent a great deal of time with John
in his hospital room. Every PIH-er visited, and so did many from
Boston's Haitian community, and his room—it had a lofty view, out
over the Charles River—was crammed full of toys. Serena set up her
apartment as a hospice, and a couple of days after John was moved
there he simply didn't wake up. Carole sat on the bed beside him and
listened, her hand on his wrist. He had Cheyne-Stokes respiration,

shallow and quick, and then a minute of apnea, and then she couldn't feel his pulse.

It seemed to me that things had turned out as well as they could have for John, under the circumstances of Haiti. PIH-ers spoke in fiery terms about those. Several said to each other, "Thank you for not letting him die *there*." Not that anyone was pleased at the outcome. The fact was the boy might have lived if he could have been extracted from Haiti sooner. But there were other consequences, surprising and consoling.

Farmer offered John's mother a job at Zanmi Lasante, and a large collection was taken up for her. Ti Fifi warned against giving her too much money at any one time, which was a good thing, an object lesson in how dangerous good intentions can be in a place as poor as Haiti. In the central plateau, word travels more quickly than most people do, and it stood to reason that a woman whose child had been flown in a jet to the United States, to *peyi kob,* "money land," would have some cash lying around. Robbers broke into her family's house outside Hinche. But thanks to Ti Fifi, there wasn't anything there worth stealing, and the thieves didn't return. As for Ti Fifi's fear that parents would besiege Zanmi Lasante with demands that their sick children be flown to Boston, too, nothing like that occurred. The next time I was in Cange, I asked Zanmi Lasante's chief handyman, Ti Jean, what the people in the region were saying about the case. He told me that everyone talked about it. "And you know what they say? They say, 'Look how much they care about us.' "

Serena had worried that this might be the last time Mass General would give one of their Haitian patients free care, but less than a month after John died, she was flying back from Haiti with another child—a little girl from a village across the reservoir from Cange with a malignant tumor on her kidney but excellent prospects and well enough to fly commercially. Mass General was waiving the cost of her care.

The staff in pediatrics had warmed up considerably to Serena and Carole. Dr. Ezekowitz especially. He was impressed at the attention they'd paid to their patient and liked to have his own staff witness it.

He sought out Serena and said, "You're a great advocate for your patient. You must be proud of yourself."

She said, "I'm not proud of myself. Patients are dying in Haiti. The mess Haiti's in is nothing to be proud of." But this was an opening she wasn't going to miss. "Dr. Ezekowitz, I would like to explore a collaborative effort. Do you think you'd like to meet Paul Farmer?"

Ezekowitz was eager to meet him, in fact. He knew of Farmer. "I think Paul is quite remarkable," he told me later. He said he thought that hospitals like Mass General had a responsibility to provide free care to patients like John. "And I think free care serves an important purpose, in that it centers people. Poverty in a place like Haiti is difficult to personalize. If it's in front of you, it has a reality."

So the meeting came off well. Farmer said, "If I might be so candid, we need help. What would you think of taking a couple of our patients a year?"

And Dr. Ezekowitz said, "Oh, I think as a minimum."

Watching the PIH-ers extract John from Cange, I had at moments, in my darkest thoughts, worried that the event might have more to do with them than with John, more to do with proving the organization's capacity for heroics than with saving a child. But then I thought: An idea like that would never have occurred to me if John had been my son. You do all you can for a patient. If I were seriously ill myself, I wouldn't find that policy unreasonable.

And yet a feeling lingered with me that the whole episode was like an object lesson in the difficulty of Farmer's enterprise, perhaps in its ultimate futility. I planned to ask him for his thoughts about the case, after a decent interval.

CHAPTER 26

It's December, two months since the medevac flight to Boston, and I'm back here with Farmer again, on the other side of the great epi divide. In the last light of the day, the outskirts of Port-au-Prince look the same to me as on every previous trip, chaotic, squalid, broken-down. For a time, driving out of the city toward the *kwazmans* of Morne Kabrit, we follow a tap-tap with some words of social commentary painted on its bumper. In translation from the Creole, they read: "Lord, a word on all this." Farmer laughs.

As he drives into the mountains, driving fast as always, the headlights bounding over ruts and boulders, I ask him how many e-mails he is receiving now. "About two hundred a day," he says. "It's still doable." Which is what he said a year ago, when he got about seventy-five a day.

He tells me, "Something's gotta give. But, as has been noted, I'm not burning out." In the light from the dashboard, I see his jaw stiffen, a momentarily pugnacious look. "And I'm not jaded either."

Once again we arrive in Cange jostled and long after dark, but without mishap—no accidents, no encounters with *zenglendo*—and Farmer gets out of his suit and into his Haiti clothes, and we sit down under the bower, dripping with vines, outside his *ti kay*. Ti Jean brings us supper and joins us.

Ti Jean is a muscular man with a wild grin, the son of a local peasant farmer. He's about thirty, old enough to have witnessed all the stages of the transformation of Cange. "It's a marvel," he says. "People were living here like pigs in a pigpen, but now you have to knock on their doors." That is, he's saying, they now *have* doors.

In addition to his role as chief handyman, Ti Jean serves as Farmer's main local male confidant. "My chief of staff," Farmer calls him. He has the right attributes. Ti Jean gives portions of his own salary to destitute patients. He has said, about National Highway 3, "I'd rather we have a fixed road and a hundred thousand extra patients a year, because it's our vocation to receive them." He has told me that if he were a *philosophe*—if, that is, his family had owned enough pigs to send him to high school—he would write a book about the Haitian bourgeoisie. An angry book, he says. He knows something about medicine and shares Farmer's scorn for notions that there's special virtue in a culture's old technologies, in the idea for instance that herbal remedies are generally to be preferred over manufactured drugs. He is also one of Farmer's chief informants on local beliefs.

To Ti Jean, animals aren't always what they seem.

"See that black dog, Polo? Was it here yesterday?"

"No."

"And did it bark twice?"

"Yes."

Ti Jean will nod knowingly. "Mmm hmmm."

In Ti Jean's cosmology, as Farmer understands it, people turn themselves into animals for shifty reasons only, or else sorcerers turn them into animals as punishment, or simply for food. Farmer interprets all this as "a giant morality play, a commentary on social inequality." He adds, "Almost invariably."

After we eat, Farmer turns on the underwater lights in his fish pond, then gazes in, naming the species. A good guest now has to join him over the fish. I say this seems to have replaced hortitorture.

"No," says Farmer, still gazing in. "It's the same as hortitorture."

Ti Jean remarks that the pond cost a lot of money, then says to Farmer, "As if I wouldn't approve. It's not one thing that makes you happy. If you only saw patients, you might not be happy."

What about all his travel? Farmer asks him.

Ti Jean allows that Farmer travels a lot. "You're like a nestless bird," he says.

"Where *is* my nest?" Farmer asks.

"Your nest is Haiti," says Ti Jean. "You go everywhere, but this is your base."

===

Of the patients I met on my previous visits, a few have long since been buried, many more have gone home, and some have stayed. A lot of the staff involved in teaching disease prevention are former patients; they tend to be zealous and they have credibility and, besides, some got sick in the first place because they were especially vulnerable. A year ago there was a family of five here all being treated for MDR. They've all been cured and have left, except for one of the sons. He believed he was responsible for infecting the rest of his family and was so extremely laden with guilt, and so neurotic about so many other things, that Farmer decided he couldn't send him away to compete for food again. So he's hired him, as a TB "outreach worker." Ti Ofa, the young man who told Farmer that he wanted to give him a chicken or a pig, has gained eight pounds since he started taking anti-AIDS drugs. The old woman who believed her son had killed his brother through sorcery has come around, after many consultations. And the lawyer Farmer hired has finally got the young security guard from Kay Epin cleared of all charges and out of jail. But in a place where medicine is still scarce, and where food is scarcer than ever and the legal system is at best rudimentary, there will always be more sorcery consults and prison extractions to come. And always more patients, of course.

Some months back, a boy named Alcante arrived at Zanmi Lasante's Children's Pavilion. Like John, he had lumps on his neck, but his were in fact symptomatic of scrofula. First-line drugs wiped out the infection. The swellings disappeared, leaving only a few small scars, and Alcante gained eight pounds, about 10 percent of his total weight. The boy was thirteen, and seemed younger because he was so small and trusting. He was the kind of child who takes strangers by the hand, and he was very beautiful looking—a perfect little body, shiny dark eyes, dimples. He changed the atmosphere in the Children's Pavilion and lessened the tightening Farmer felt in his chest as he climbed the stairs to that wing. For Farmer, the children's ward contained Zanmi Lasante's most harrowing sights and painful ghosts, and I think Alcante came to seem like the guardian angel of the place, or like Farmer's. He kept the boy in Cange several weeks longer than necessary. He called him "a P.O.P."—a prisoner of Paul. Finally, he sent him home.

As a rule, a child with scrofula gets it from a close contact, usually the mother or father. So one of Zanmi Lasante's community health workers brought the rest of Alcante's family to Cange—they were "trolled in," as Farmer puts it. Several had TB, including Alcante's father, who is still in therapy. Now Farmer wants to see for himself what home means to Alcante. He plans to hike to their homestead. "The family is so afflicted," he explains, then adds, "Some people would say this is a scattershot approach. We would answer, 'Not at all. It's through journeys to the sick that we identify needs and problems.' "

Alcante lives in a town called Casse. The hike is longer than the first long one I took with Farmer to Morne Michel, but the trails aren't as steep. This is what he told me last night. So I have only a vague idea of how many hours the trip will take, until we're walking out the front gate and Ti Jean, who is coming with us, asks if I have brought my flashlight.

I haven't. I offer to go back for it. Farmer doesn't think I should. Inevitably, some emergency will have cropped up, and going back will get him entangled in it. Delay now will mean further delay. Farmer is wearing a baseball cap, which looks a few sizes too large, and for a moment I imagine him a gawky teenager on the way to a ball game with his dad. His thin frame and the shininess of his face make this possible, and also a quality of innocence that surfaces at times—he's apt, for example, in the midst of an erudite discourse on the economic distribution of infectious disease, to startle you by interjecting, eagerly, "Ask me a question about *Lord of the Rings*." He's reread those books again and again over the years since he was eleven. But now he's leading the way out of Zanmi Lasante, in every sense the man in charge, and I realize I'm not worried about the flashlight. This strikes me as unusual. I've never found it easy to trust another person to lead me anywhere, but I trust Farmer.

We head off along dirt paths etched into the sides of the hills beside the Péligre Reservoir, and soon I'm scrambling up the eroded face of a cliff. I'm drenched with sweat by the time we get to the top, where Farmer is waiting for me. I'm reminded of the epic hike to Morne Michel. As we go on, Farmer calls back over his shoulder—his voice makes it plain he's joking—that if I have chest pains, I should tell him right away. I take a long swig of water as we stride across a ridge through yellow grass, Farmer pointing out "the peculiarly steep and conical hill" on which he sat in solitude years ago, writing *AIDS and Accusation.*

Ti Jean is carrying a large water jug, filled from a tap at the medical complex. It's potable water. Farmer and Ti Jean have immunity to whatever microorganisms it contains, but American visitors who drink it often come down with bowel troubles, not dangerously but uncomfortably. So I've brought my own jug of filtered water, but it isn't very large. By the time we make our first stop, I've drunk half, and Ti Jean and Farmer and Zanmi Lasante's pharmacist, who is also coming along, haven't even opened their jug.

Farmer has planned an intermediate house call on the way to Alcante's home in Casse. Somewhere in the mountains, we stop at a hut—two tiny rooms, dirt floors, a roof of banana fronds, pro-Aristide posters on the walls, and an elderly-looking couple sitting together on a straw mat. Farmer has brought along the man's medical records. He sits down on a chair near the doorway and reads aloud from them. "Since 1989 he's been coming to ZL and he's been getting antihypertensives. I saw him last in 1997 and he had malaria and then it says, 'Come back Thursday for a follow-up.' He didn't come back. And oops, here we go, it says here, 'Trouble standing up.' And his son had come for medicine for his blood pressure." Farmer kneels on the dirt floor and takes the man's pulse and blood pressure, then puts on a stethoscope and listens to his chest for a while. Cocks crow outside.

The air inside is still and hot, vibrating with flies. The old man says he felt a little pain at the center of his chest and afterward weakness in his legs. Farmer says to me, "I know what I'm going to do. Get his blood pressure down to normal, then get him two Canadian crutches. I think he probably had a stroke, but he should be able to recover is what I'm saying. His deficit is *minimal.* So I have to get somebody to help me get the Canadian crutches here. To get his blood pressure just right would be easy at the Brigham. It's not easy here, and how do we check and make sure he's doing his physical therapy?"

The old man's wife says she wants her blood pressure checked, too. Kneeling beside her, Farmer says in English, "She's sixty-two. Going on a hundred," adding, as if to himself, "We are far from the Brigham, my friend." The woman's pressure is high, too, he says. I, meanwhile, am trying to think of what Farmer said to me a year ago about the profound difference between being bedridden in a nice house outside Boston and mat-ridden in a hut like this, but I can't stop thinking at the same time about the little pain that has been flitting around behind my left nipple, on and off ever since that first cliff climb.

Finally, I tell Farmer about the pain. Then I apologize, and he says, "Don't be silly. Tell me more about it." He asks me a dozen questions, and says he thinks I just have heartburn. "But if it gets worse, you have to tell me. You don't want to see Alcante that bad. Promise?"

Several small children have come to the doorway. They stand there, peering in. Farmer says to them, speaking of the sad-looking woman of the house, "You love her a lot? Do you tell her? Don't lie to me now." The children giggle. The old woman smiles. Farmer nods toward a naked toddler in the doorway. "Look at his toy."

The child is sucking the thumb of one hand. In the other, he holds a piece of coarse hemp string. A rock is tied to the end of it.

"Rocks 'R' Us," says Farmer, and I laugh. I can't stop. Farmer starts laughing, too, saying, "Now *I'm* going to have chest pain. God is going to strike me dead." He says that he's going to give me half a beta-blocker just in case, and still I can't stop laughing.

"God is going to strike me dead," he says again. "For drinking more than my share of water, for not living humbly, for my *bad* sense of humor. It's your fault. I'm playing to my audience."

But, I think, he hasn't drunk any water yet.

He gives the couple their pills and instructions. Good-byes are always long in Haiti. When we get outside, Farmer says, "This was a *bel kout nas,* a good cast of the net. We came to see Papa and got Grandma, too. Just in time. Before she got run over by a reindeer."

I've heard him use the fishing metaphor many times. When a sick person is discovered by accident, he usually says he's made a lucky catch. As if Zanmi Lasante didn't have enough patients already.

"Is there a long way still to go?" I ask, as we walk on.

"Oh, yeah! This is a quarter of the way there."

"A quarter?"

Since the death of the boy John, I've been trying to form my question for Farmer about that case. I remember a remark he made to me a year ago in these hills: "You *should* compare suffering. Which suffering is worse. It's called triage."

The term comes from the fourteenth-century French *trier,* "to pick or cull," and was first used to describe the sorting of wool according to its quality. In modern medical usage, *triage* has two different meanings, nearly opposite. In situations where doctors and nurses and tools are limited, on battlefields, for instance, one performs triage by attending first to the severely wounded who have the best chance of survival. The aim is to save as many as possible; the others may have to die unattended. In the peacetime case, however, in well-staffed and well-stocked American emergency rooms, for example, *triage* isn't supposed to imply withholding care from anyone; rather, it's identifying the patients in gravest danger and giving them priority.

Farmer has constructed his life around this second kind of triage. What else is a "preferential option for the poor" in medicine? But Haiti more nearly resembles a battlefield than a place at peace. Walking behind him, I say there must always be situations here where the choice to do one necessary thing also means the choice not to do another—not just to defer the other but not to do it.

"All the time," he says.

"Throughout your whole career you've had to face this, right?"

"Yes. I do it every day. Do this instead of that. Every day all day long, that's all I do. Is not do things."

So, I ask, what about the case of John? What about the twenty thousand dollars that PIH spent on the medevac flight to get him out of Haiti? Not long after John died, a PIH-er, a relatively new one, said to me that she couldn't help thinking of all the things they could have done with that twenty thousand dollars. What is his response to that? "I don't mean this at all critically," I add, hurrying along behind him.

"Come on," he says over his shoulder. "I'm not hypersensitive. But we've already discussed this, so many times. I'm just failing to do a good job or you're not convinced. Maybe I'll never convince you that the choices we make are good ones."

I don't want to nettle him. For one thing, he's both my guide and my doctor for today. But I recognize his tone of voice. He's not really irritated. He's just delivering a preamble, warming up his argument.

He continues, talking over his shoulder to me as we walk on. "Let me say a couple of things about this particular case, if you like. One is, remember of course that John was referred to Boston as dying of a treatable tumor, a very rare tumor. He wasn't referred to Mass General before we knew what he had. So when he was referred, it was for free care because he had such a rare thing and it was treatable, and the predicted cure rate was sixty to seventy percent. All right. Good enough. That was what the decision was made on. And there was no way for us to find out that John didn't have locally invasive disease without metastases, because it required a diagnostic test that we can't do here. So the other thing is, the bottom line is, why do we intervene as aggressively as we can with that kid and not with another? Because his mother brought him to us and that's where he was, in our clinic."

"I wondered when Serena and Carole came to get him, if you'd have decided to bring him after all, if you'd been there. He was so emaciated."

"The emaciation wouldn't have stopped me. If I'd seen him and seen how far he'd gone downhill, I wouldn't have stopped the process.

Why? On what grounds? We didn't know until he got to Boston that the cancer had invaded his vertebrae."

We climb another cliff, and I am breathing too hard to speak. After a short pause, he says, "I have to tell you, though, I'm a little troubled by these comments from the new PIH-er. Because I have to *work* with these people. The last thing I want to do is expend my energy trying to convince my own co-workers. Now I have to, of course. But I don't like it. The Haitians have a lot to say about inviting the wrong people into your midst, you know."

"I don't want to misrepresent it," I say. "Your PIH-er wasn't saying you shouldn't have brought John to Boston. Only that it was a shame you had to spend so much, given what else you could do with twenty grand."

"Yeah, but there are so many ways of saying that," he replies. "For example, why didn't the airplane company that makes money, the mercenaries, why didn't they pay for his flight? That's a way of saying it. Or how about this way? How about if I say, I have fought for *my whole life* a long defeat. How about that? How about if I said, That's all it adds up to is defeat?"

"A long defeat."

"I have fought the long defeat and brought other people on to fight the long defeat, and I'm not going to stop because we keep losing. Now I actually think sometimes we may *win*. I don't dislike victory. You and I have discussed this so many times."

"Sorry."

"No, no, I'm not complaining," he says. "You know, people from our background—like you, like most PIH-ers, like me—we're used to being on a victory team, and actually what we're really trying to do in PIH is to make common cause with the *losers*. Those are two very different things. We *want* to be on the winning team, but at the *risk* of turning our backs on the losers, no, it's not worth it. So you fight the long defeat." He pauses. "How you feelin'? Is that chest pain gone?"

I am overheated, but that little flitting pain hasn't come again.

Farmer continues, "And most of the time when people ask about triage, most of the time they're asking not with open hostility but deep distrust of our answer. They already have the answer. And that of course is the energy-draining process, because you understand that a substantial proportion of the questions are asked in a, you know, in a very, what's the word?"

"With an animus?"

"Yeah."

He's silent as we scrabble down a hilly section of the trail. At the bottom, he resumes. "The salary of a first-world doctor. How about that? Talk about all the money that could have been spent on other things, what about a doctor's salary?"

I laugh. "I hadn't thought of that."

"Well, of course. See, the truly humble think of that before they say the other. I'm not truly humble. I'm trying to be humble. So let me ask you another question. What is it that makes people not think that? Why doesn't a young American doctor say, 'Gee, my salary is five times what John's airplane ride cost. And I'm twenty-nine or thirty-some years old.' If you say that stuff out loud, you sound like an ass-hole. Whereas if you say the other stuff, you just sound thoughtful. Now what's wrong with that? What's wrong with this picture? If you say, Well, I just think how much could have been done with twenty thousand dollars, you sound thoughtful, sensible, you know, reason-able, rational, someone you really want on your side. However, if you were to point out, *But* a young attending physician makes *one hundred thousand* dollars, not twenty, and that's *five* times what it cost to try to save a boy's life—that just makes you sound like an asshole. Same world, same numbers, same figures, same currency. It's just, you know, I never have been able to figure it out. I mean, I've figured it out, but I realize now it takes *so much time* to get to that point, to explain it, without offending someone. So what are you thinkin'?"

"I like the line about the long defeat," I tell him.

"I would regard that as the basic stance of O for the P," he replies. "I don't care if we lose, I'm gonna try to do the right thing."

"But you're going to try to win."

"Of course! We're not, you know, masochistic. And then all the victories are gravy, you know? The other option is to be jaded because you've been fighting a defeat for eighteen years, and trying to stop it, at least save the elbow joint for Kenol, you know." He's referring to a current patient, a boy back in Cange whose hand got caught in a sugar-cane press—a "low medieval device," Farmer called it—and ended up with gangrene. In the end, his arm had to be amputated above the elbow joint. (After the operation, he said he wanted a radio. Farmer bought him one on his latest Miami day. Zanmi Lasante will send him to school.)

"How's your chest?" Farmer asks.

It feels all right, in fact. But there is only one mouthful of water left in my jug, and Farmer has said he'd prefer that I not drink the unfil-tered water Ti Jean is carrying. So, for the moment, I think I'd rather be thirsty.

Farmer goes on, "If we could identify losers like John, and not waste our time and energy on them, then we'd be all good, as they say in the States. Right? But the point of O for the P is that you never do that. You never risk that. Because before you turn your back on some-one like John you have to be really really sure, and the more you learn about John's family the more you realize that the whole family, their whole— I mean, they're basically extinct, right? He was the last kid. They're extinct. His mother's bloodline is just gone. It sounds Dar-winian, but you know what I mean. Shit, man, how can you be an O for the P doc and be willing to take that risk without all the data you can get? Every patient is a sign. Every patient is a test. Like this guy we just saw. The guy's living in dirt, the guy who needs Canadian crutches? You realize how much shit I'd get for that, Canadian crutches in rural Haiti?"

"Because they're not appropriate technology?"

"Yeah. Now you can see the critiques revealed for what they are. But I have to limit the amount of time I put into explaining all that or it just sucks your soul dry. If I spent all my time arguing, No, this man needs Canadian crutches *and* a roof *and* a floor. I mean, if you're only defensive. If you say, Fuck you, man, I already *built* a thousand houses in this country, how many have you built? That doesn't go anywhere either. But that's the very doctor they'd be criticizing, one who's already done his housing fellowship and his practicum in blah blah blah. If you spend all your time arguing about that stuff, defending yourself, you don't get your work done. It must mean *something* that Ti Jean doesn't talk about things like appropriate technology."

We are walking, Farmer has said, through what used to be rebel territory, during both Haiti's slave days and the years when the U.S. Marines occupied the country. It seems different from the areas near Cange. The farmyards and even the hilltops look a little more fertile, a little less bereft of soil and trees. But the land is just as crowded. We have been trudging through deep country, far from anything that could even be called a road, and yet there's hardly been a moment when other people haven't been in sight or just around the next turn in the trail.

We've forded one big river—pigs rooting in the banks, chunks of earth falling into the water, and irrationally, I felt as though I should catch the soil in my arms and put it back. I'm not sure how many hours we've been walking. It must be at least four. We've crossed ridge after ridge, and we're still encountering the works of PIH. Some are inanimate—a school that Zanmi Lasante built out here in the mountains—but mostly they're patients. I've lost count of their numbers, and we're still running into them. There are the fairly healthy-looking ones who say to Farmer in Creole, "Hi, my Doc," or "How's my Doc's little body today?" And patients who are works in progress. The most memorable for me is a girl whose neck and chest were burned some time ago. It looks as if the flesh on the lower part of her face had melted and then hardened into a beard of skin, the strands of the beard attaching her jaw and chin to her chest and shoulders more and more tightly as she's grown. Never mind the grotesque scarring, in another year or so, her mouth will be pulled permanently open. Unless she gets to a plastic surgeon. Farmer has been trying to arrange the necessary operations in the United States. "It's a *bwat*," he says.

"We getting close to Casse?" I ask.

"Well, you don't want to know just yet." He smiles. He stops and points to a hilltop in the distance. "Wait'll we get over that ridge. Then I'll break it to you. Khyber Pass. Ruby Ridge. I'm sorry. *Lord of the Rings,* Redhorn Pass. Smell this. It's campêche."

I drank my last sip of water some time ago, and I'm feeling slightly dizzy as we continue on. My mouth has grown so dry that I croak when I try to speak.

Farmer has noticed. He starts calling out, "Do you have oranges?" at every farmyard we pass. I end up sitting with my back against a tree, devouring six oranges, one right after the other. And when we finally reach Casse, a brown and dusty, dirt-street market town, constructed of wood and corrugated metal, Farmer feeds me Cokes.

"I can't tell you how much better I feel."

"Hydration," he says.

Zanmi Lasante's local health worker—a barefoot woman in a dress—shows us the way to Alcante's house. (Farmer waited for her to find us. He didn't ask the strangers in Casse for directions. "Because they're Hats, there would be no shortage of wrong answers. You learn that in year three or four.") Another half hour's walk and we arrive at the farm, which consists of a stand of millet, a cook shack with a three-rocks fireplace, and a hut made of what is known as wattle and daub— that is, dried mud and sticks. The roof is old banana bark, patched all over with rags.

"Alcante!" says Farmer. "I'm happy to see you."

"And I'm delighted to see you!" says the shiny little boy. He calls to his sisters, emerging from the hut, "Are there any more chairs here? We need more chairs."

"The little social director," Farmer says to me. "He's just so . . ." His voice trails off. He grins.

Alcante's father was shaving when we arrived—with a painted shard of glass for a mirror and a razor blade and no soap or water. He finishes the job. Gradually, the rest of the family emerges from the hut, and I am reminded of the routine at the circus in which an apparently endless stream of people comes out of a tiny car. I estimate the hut to be about ten feet by twenty, and I count ten souls who live in it. Farmer gazes at the hut. "Well, I guess I don't need to do a house inspection." He stares at it some more. "On a scale of one to ten, this is a one."

A long chat ensues. From it Farmer draws a variety of lessons for me. Of the several cases of TB in this family, only the father's was detectable by sputum smear. That is, his was the only case that involved the lungs and was contagious, the only epidemiologically significant case, the only kind of case that DOTS addresses. "So here's a house full of TB, where you only have one case according to the DOTS system," says Farmer. "The rest had extrapulmonary disease, which doesn't count. It can kill ya but it doesn't count." He adds, and for a moment he is back in Peru, "We never wanted to get rid of *las normas,* we just wanted to extend them, and add some flexibility."

There's also a sociopolitical lesson to draw, of course: "Look at Alcante's family. It's intact, the kids are bright and clever, and the father can't walk. And they just can't make it. It's fucking unfair. The woman who said to me years ago, Are you incapable of complexity? That was an epiphany for me. Are you going to punish people for thinking TB comes from sorcery? It's like the guy on our own team, a nice guy, who said he would help with a water project in a town here, but only if the people really showed they wanted it. What if that standard had been applied to me when I was a kid, before I knew that water could carry organisms that made people sick?"

He concludes the dismount, saying, "I'm glad we came, because now we know how grim it is and we can intervene aggressively."

I know what this means: a new house with a concrete floor and metal roof, further arrangements for improving the family's nutrition, school tuition for the kids. Here's a good deed in progress, and a perfect example of the Farmer method. First, you perform what he calls "the distal intervention" and cure the family of TB. Then you start changing the conditions that made them especially vulnerable to TB in the first place.

I am aware of other voices that would praise a trip like this for its good intentions, and yet describe it as an example of what is wrong with Farmer's approach. Here's an influential anthropologist, medical diplomat, public health administrator, epidemiologist, who has helped to bring new resolve and hope to some of the world's most dreadful problems, and he's just spent seven hours making house calls. How many desperate families live in Haiti? He's made this trip to visit two.

I think of the wealthy friend of Howard Hiatt's who balked at contributing to PIH because, while he knew about Farmer's work in Haiti and considered it impressive, he doubted anyone could reproduce it. I've heard variations on that theme. Farmer and Kim do things that no one else can do. Zanmi Lasante won't survive Farmer. Partners In Health is an organization that relies too much on a genius. All the serious, sympathetic critiques come down to these two arguments: Hiking into the hills to see just one patient or two is a dumb way for Farmer to spend his time, and even if it weren't, not many other people will follow his example, not enough to make much difference in the world.

But standard notions of efficiency, notions about cost-effectiveness, about big people performing big jobs, haven't worked so well themselves. Long ago in North Carolina, Farmer watched the nuns doing menial chores on behalf of migrant laborers, and in the years since he's come to think that a willingness to do what he calls "unglamorous scut work" is the secret to successful projects in places like Cange and Carabayllo. "And," he says, "another secret: a reluctance to do scut work is why a lot of my peers don't stick with this kind of work." In public health projects in difficult locales, theory often outruns practice. Individual patients get forgotten, and what seems like a small problem gets ignored, until it grows large, like MDR. "If you focus on individual patients," Jim Kim says, "you can't get sloppy."

That approach has worked for PIH. And I can imagine Farmer saying he doesn't care if no one else is willing to follow their example. He's still going to make these hikes, he'd insist, because if you say that seven hours is too long to walk for two families of patients, you're saying that their lives matter less than some others', and the idea that some lives matter less is the root of all that's wrong with the world. I think he undertakes what, earlier today, he called "journeys to the sick" in part because he has to, in order to keep going. "That's when I feel most alive," he told me once on an airplane, "when I'm helping people." He makes these house calls regularly and usually without *blan* witnesses, at times when no one from Harvard or WHO can see him kneeling on mud floors with his stethoscope plugged in. This matters to him, I think—to feel, at least occasionally, that he doctors in obscurity, so that he knows he doctors first of all because he believes it's the right thing to do.

If you do the right thing well, you avoid futility. His patients tend to get better. They all get comforted. And he carries off, among other things, images of them and their medieval huts. These refresh his passion and authority, so that he can travel a quarter of a million miles a year and scheme and write about the health of populations. Doctoring is the ultimate source of his power, I think. His basic message is simple: This person is sick, and I am a doctor. Everyone, potentially, can understand and sympathize, since everyone knows or imagines sickness personally. And it can't be hard for most people to imagine what it would be like to have no doctor, no hope of medicine. I think Farmer taps into a universal anxiety and also into a fundamental place in some troubled consciences, into what he calls "ambivalence," the often unacknowledged uneasiness that some of the fortunate feel about their place in the world, the thing he once told me he designed his life to avoid.

"The best thing about Paul is those hikes," Ophelia says. "You have to believe that small gestures matter, that they do add up." Earlier today Farmer said that he'd brought on others to fight "the long defeat." The numbers are impressive. They include priests and nuns and professors and secretaries and businessmen and church ladies and peasants like Ti Jean and also dozens of medical students and doctors, who have enlisted to work in places such as Cange and Siberia and the slums of Lima. Some of the students and doctors work for nothing, some earn much less than they could elsewhere, some raise their own salaries through grants. I once heard Farmer say that he hoped a day would come when he could do a good job just by showing up. It seems to me that time has already arrived. A great deal of what he's started goes on without him now, in Roxbury and Tomsk and Peru and, some of the year, in Haiti. Meanwhile, other definitions than the usual, of what can be done and what is reasonable to do in medicine and public health, have spread from him. They're still spreading, like ripples in a pond.

How does one person with great talents come to exert a force on the world? I think in Farmer's case the answer lies somewhere in the apparent craziness, the sheer impracticality, of half of everything he does, including the hike to Casse.

══

We still have to get back to Zanmi Lasante. The sun is setting by the time we finally leave Alcante's family. Gray clouds billow over the mountains we crossed earlier today. "The westering sun is rebuking us," says Farmer.

He and Ti Jean confer. They decide we can't walk back the way we came, not across rivers and over steep paths in the dark, without a flashlight. What they mean is they don't think I'd make it. I'm not pleased that they think this but am relieved that they do. We arrive back in Casse around dusk. An old man rides down the dirt street on a horse, then a young man on a motorbike, whom Farmer stops. He asks the driver if he'll give one of our party, the pharmacist, a lift to Cange, and the young man says he will, but for a hundred dollars. "What's your name?" says Farmer in Creole.

"Jackie," he replies. Then he asks, "Are you Doktè Paul?"

"Yes. We know your machine eats gas and we'll replace it. We brought some money for a family here, and they are living in squalor, unlike you, Jackie. And if you get sick, I won't ask you for a hundred dollars."

A little crowd has gathered to listen in. Now everyone, including Jackie, laughs. So it's settled. The pharmacist will ride with Jackie back to Cange and send a truck for Ti Jean and Farmer and me. Farmer didn't even break a sweat in the previous hours of walking, and now he feels like walking some more. ("Everyone thinks I'm unhealthy," he says to me. "In fact? Healthy as a horse.") So we won't wait in Casse for the truck. Ti Jean and Farmer and I will walk along the dirt road that leads from Casse to Thomonde, the route the truck will have to take.

We stroll out of the village in fading light. The air is merely warm now, the kind of air that I'll remember on winter nights in northern places and think I must have dreamed. Soon, there being no electrical lights for miles and miles in any direction, the stars pop out en masse, bright enough, it seems, to faintly light the road. "This is nice," Farmer says to me. "A break from my clinic, from airplanes. I know your feet hurt, but I do in many ways prefer walking." A cozy feeling seems to spread from him. It's as if we're three kids out after bedtime and we can say whatever is really on our minds but don't have to. I sing a snatch of an army marching song. "You had a good home but you left."

"You had a nice bus but you left," sings Farmer.

Roosters crow in the night. Now and then a dog barks. Then we hear a strange sound coming toward us, like something scraping the road. "What is it?" Farmer asks Ti Jean.

Ti Jean says, *"Job pa-l."* The literal translation is: "Its own job." He means, "Don't ask." In a moment, the shapes of a pair of men appear, dragging some sawn lumber down the road toward Casse. A few minutes later we hear a squeaking sound approaching. Farmer asks Ti Jean what it is, and Ti Jean answers more emphatically. *"Zafè bounda-l!"* Which means, "Its own ass!" That is, he's telling Farmer to shut up and mind his own business. A moment later the shape of a person on a squeaky old bicycle passes in the starlight.

This continues. Another figure passes us, and Farmer says, *"Bonsoir,"* and Ti Jean shushes him, then issues these instructions: If someone passes you at night and doesn't speak, you too must remain silent, but if the person asks who you are, you must say, "I am who you are," and if the person asks what you do, you must say, "I do what you do."

What's the danger? Farmer asks.

Ti Jean says you might be talking to a demon who will steal your spirit. Then you'll wake up in the morning with diarrhea and vomiting, and the doctor will say you have typhoid or malaria, but in fact the problem will be more complex. "You should take the medicines," says Ti Jean. "But then you should also go to a Voodoo priest."

We stroll on. Farmer says that Ti Jean's discourse has reminded him of his first ardent explorations of Haiti and of the dozens of Voodoo ceremonies he attended. Contrary to almost everything he'd read about their luridness, he found them long and boring. "The majority were held because someone was sick." He asks Ti Jean his opinion. Are half of Voodoo ceremonies attempts to drive away illness?

"Three-quarters," says Ti Jean.

"Isn't it amazing," Farmer says to me, "that this simple fact has eluded all the many commentaries on Voodoo?"

We've walked three hours from Casse, eleven hours in all today, when I finally feel as though I can't go any farther. When I say so, Farmer calls a halt. I'm grateful that he doesn't tease me. We sit down on the side of the lumpy dirt road, on the crest of a hill, facing east. I have a candy bar, and we share it like a trio of Boy Scouts under the stars. Ti Jean points out a blinking red light far away, a radio tower across the border in the Dominican Republic. Staring at it, I hear Farmer's voice beside me, his gentle doctor's voice, asking how I feel. I tell him the truth—tired but feeling fine. And then, clear of all his duties for now, his last patient of the day attended to, he lies back on the ground and stares at the stars. "There's Orion's belt . . ."

From somewhere in the valley below us comes the sound of drums. I recall the time I spent here in the central plateau with the American soldiers, and I remember the sound of Voodoo drums wafting into the army barracks in Mirebalais at night and how unsettling it was to some of us sitting there, in all its mystery. I'm sure we'd have felt different if we'd known we were probably hearing ceremonies to cure the sick. For myself, right now, I like the sound, like so many hearts beating through a single stethoscope.

In June 2002, seven years after the death of Father Jack Roussin, WHO adopted new prescriptions for dealing with MDR-TB, virtually the same as PIH had used in Carabayllo. For Jim Kim this marked the end of a long campaign. "The world changed yesterday," he wrote from Geneva to all of PIH. The prices of second-line antibiotics continued to decline, and the drugs now flowed fairly smoothly through the Green Light Committee to, among other places, Peru, where about 1,000 chronic patients were either cured or in treatment. About 250 were receiving the drugs in Tomsk, and, largely because of the efforts of WHO, the Russian Ministry of Health had finally agreed to the terms of the World Bank's TB loan—150 million dollars to begin to fight the epidemic throughout the country.

The twin pandemics of AIDS and tuberculosis raged on, of course, magnifying each other, in Africa and Asia, eastern Europe and Latin America. Mathematical models predicted widening global catastrophe—100 million HIV infections in the world by the year 2010. Some prominent voices, some in the U.S. government, still argued that AIDS could not be treated in desperately impoverished places. But this view seemed to be fading. The prices of antiretrovirals were falling, even more dramatically than the prices of second-line TB drugs. This was thanks to a growing worldwide campaign for treating AIDS wherever it occurred. Jim Kim had often said that the world's response to AIDS and TB would define the moral standing of his generation. In 2003, a new director general took over at WHO, and he asked Jim to serve as his senior adviser. Meanwhile, the example of Zanmi Lasante was growing, and Cange had become a favorite destination for global health policy makers and American politicians.

The Global Fund money was delayed, as such monies often are, but Farmer chose not to wait, and in the summer of 2002 the expansion of Zanmi Lasante began—the expansion of the entire system, including antiretroviral treatment, throughout the central plateau. To pay the bills until the Global Fund money arrived, PIH borrowed $2 million from a commercial bank in Boston—Tom White guaranteed the loan and soon paid off a part of it, and the PIH employees with the highest salaries took care of interest payments on the rest. In essence, Farmer's plan was to "beef up" the health facilities in the central plateau, first of all in towns near Cange. He dispatched teams of Haitian and American doctors and technicians to three towns. One team went to a settlement called Lascahobas, some miles north of Cange. When they arrived, they found a wretched, nearly empty private hospital and a nearly empty public clinic, which had almost no drugs on hand, unreliable electrical power for a few hours a day, and a staff of one doctor and five nurses who all went home for good at 1:00 P.M. Serena Koenig, a member of the Lascahobas team, described the situation as "a nightmare." But by October, after a month of beefing up, that clinic had a generator, a lab, a full supply of medicines, and doctors on hand all day. And the place was packed with patients, about two hundred daily, sometimes three hundred. The decline in foreign aid to Haiti and to the Haitian government continued, and so did the flood of patients to Cange. But not many came from Lascahobas anymore. The passenger truck from there to Zanmi Lasante, which used to be completely filled, had stopped making the run for lack of riders.

Haiti was still bleeding away, like its topsoil. The whole situation was "rotten," Farmer wrote. He added, "But there are some spots of hope." With help from Ti Fifi, a group of Cangeois had drafted a petition to President Aristide asking for electricity. By late October, pylons were being erected to carry power from the dam at Péligre to Cange for a few hours a day. And the Red Cross had announced plans to establish a transfusion post at Zanmi Lasante. Nearly twenty years since

Farmer had watched a woman die in Léogâne for lack of a transfusion, and he finally had a blood bank that could serve the central plateau, a source of blood that patients wouldn't have to pay for. "No more weeping over blood," he wrote to me.

Some of his e-mails were ebullient: "We're growing by leaps and bounds." Zanmi Lasante's staff now included more than two hundred community health workers, about a dozen nurses, and twelve doctors, among them a Cuban surgeon and a Cuban pediatrician. They were caring for more than three thousand HIV patients, and providing anti-retrovirals to about 350. They now had the equipment and trained personnel to do some of their own high-tech AIDS diagnostics. Meanwhile, Père Lafontant had managed the construction of a second operating room. Also in 2002, Cange saw its first open-heart surgeries, performed by teams from the Brigham and South Carolina. I felt tempted to ask Farmer if this was appropriate technology—not to hear the answer, just to hear him say it.

ACKNOWLEDGMENTS

I feel grateful to all the people who appear in this book, and especially to Jaime Bayona, Ophelia Dahl, Howard Hiatt, Jim Yong Kim, and Tom White. I feel grateful beyond measure to Paul Farmer and, I must say, to the fates that allowed my path to cross his.

I want to thank my editors, Kate Medina and Richard Todd, who supported this project, encouraged me, and lent painstaking editorial assistance. My thanks to John Bennet, Ann Goldstein, Marina Harss, and David Remnick at *The New Yorker;* to the writers Stuart Dybek, Jonathan Harr, Craig Nova, John O'Brien, and Doug Whynott; to Fran, Nat, and Alice; and to Georges Borchardt, Evan Camfield, Benjamin Dreyer, Amy Edelman, John Graiff, Jamie Kilbreth, Jessica Kirshner, and Michael Siegel.

I want to express my gratitude to Didi and Catherine Farmer, to Jorge Pérez, to Serena Koenig and Carole Smarth, to the brilliant and lovely Mercedes Becerra, and to all the other members, past and present, of Partners In Health, especially the following: Ania Barciak, Donna Barry, Heidi Behforouz, Arachu Castro, Chris Douglas, Elizabeth Foley, Ken Fox, Hamish Fraser, Nicole Gastineau, Melissa Gillooly, Raj Gupta, Ann Hyson, Keith Joseph, Kathryn Kempton, Kedar Mate, Ellen Meltzer, Joyce Millen, Carole Mitnick, Mark Moseley, Joia Mukherjee, Kristin Nelson, Denise Payne, Michael Rich, Cynthia Rose, Aaron Shakow, Jenn Singler, Mary Kay Smith-Fawzi, Laura Tarter, Chris Vanderwarker, David Walton, and Michelle Welshhans. I wish to thank Gene Bukhman, Ed Nardell, and Peter

Small for speaking to me about drug resistance in tuberculosis and other related matters. I am in debt to many others as well: John Ayanian, Ethan Canin, Jennie LaBalme, Anne McCormack, Todd McCormack, Haun Saussy, and Jackie Williams for sharing their reminiscences and insight; Leon Eisenberg, Byron Good, and Arthur Kleinman for talking to me about Paul Farmer's student years and subsequent career; Guido Bakker and Richard Laing for helpful discussions about drugs and drug pricing; Liam Harte and Aaron Shakow for discussions about utilitarian philosophy and cost-effectiveness; Christine Collins for a tour of the Brigham; Elena Osso for helping to show me Carabayllo; Aryeh Neier for discussing the background of the Open Society Institute's work on TB in Russia; Arata Kochi and J. W. Lee of WHO, also Mario Raviglione for long, pleasant conversations in Geneva; Jamie Maguire and Marshall Wolf for discussing Paul Farmer's medical career with me; Julius Richmond for many long chats about PIH and international health; Michael Iseman for an interview about Paul Farmer's work and for correcting some of my misconceptions about tuberculosis; the lovely Oksana Ponomarenko for making my trip to Siberia possible, and Tim Healing, Sasha Pasechnikov, and Sasha Trusov for helping to make it informative and congenial; Bill Foege and Mark Rosenberg for discussing a wide range of matters.

I wish to offer special thanks to Oaksook Kim, and to the extended Farmer family—especially Ginny, Katy, Jeff, Jennifer, and Peggy—for sharing their memories, for their hospitality, for their warmth.

I have changed the names of some of the Haitian citizens I depicted and have omitted the surnames of some others. The reason is simple: the possibility of a return to systematic, violent political repression in Haiti and with it more cases like that of "Chouchou Louis." For their extraordinary grace and kindness, I offer my thanks to all the workers and patients whom I met at Zanmi Lasante, including "Ti Fifi," Dr. Fernet Léandre, Dr. Hugo Jérôme, Ti Jean, and, of course, Fritz and Mamito and Flore Lafontant.

SELECTED BIBLIOGRAPHY

The following is a list—complete as of May 2003—of the published writings of Paul Edward Farmer.

BOOKS

Farmer, P. E. *AIDS and Accusation: Haiti and the Geography of Blame.* Berkeley: University of California Press, 1992.

———. *The Uses of Haiti.* Monroe, Maine: Common Courage Press, 1994. (Second edition published in 2002.)

———. *¿Haití para qué?* Hondarribia, Spain: HIRU Argitaletxea, 1994.

———. *Sida en Haïti: La victime accusée.* Paris: Editions Karthala, 1996.

———. *Infections and Inequalities: The Modern Plagues.* Berkeley: University of California Press, 1999. (Second edition published in 2001.)

———. *Pathologies of Power: Health, Human Rights, and the New War on the Poor.* Berkeley: University of California Press, 2002.

BOOKS EDITED

Farmer, P. E., Connors, M., Simmons, J. (eds.). *Women, Poverty, and AIDS: Sex, Drugs, and Structural Violence.* Monroe, Maine: Common Courage Press, 1996.

BOOK CHAPTERS

Daily, J., Farmer, P. E., Rhatigan, J., Katz, J., Furin, J. J. Women and HIV infection. In Farmer, P. E., Connors, M., Simmons, J. (eds.). *Women, Poverty, and AIDS: Sex, Drugs, and Structural Violence.* Monroe, Maine: Common Courage Press, 1996:125–144.

Farmer, P. E. AIDS and accusation: Haiti, Haitians and the geography of blame. In Feldman, D. (ed.). *AIDS and Culture: The Human Factor.* New York: Praeger Scientific, 1990:122–150.

————. Birth of the *klinik:* The making of Haitian professional psychiatry. In Gaines, A. (ed.). *Ethnopsychiatry.* Albany: State University of New York Press, 1992:251–272.

————. New disorder, old dilemmas: AIDS and anthropology in Haiti. In Herdt, G., Lindenbaum, S. (eds.). *The Time of AIDS.* Los Angeles: Sage, 1992:287–318.

————. Culture, poverty, and the dynamics of HIV transmission in rural Haiti. In Brummelhuis, H. T., Herdt, G. (eds.). *Culture and Sexual Risk: Anthropological Perspectives on AIDS.* Newark, N.J.: Gordon and Breach, 1995:3–28.

————. Pestilence and restraint: Haitians, Guantánamo, and the logic of quarantine. In Hannaway, C., Harden, V. A., Parascandola, J. (eds.). *AIDS and the Public Debate: Historical and Contemporary Perspectives.* Burke, Va.: IOS Press, 1995:139–152.

————. The significance of Haiti. In North American Congress on Latin America (ed.). *Haiti: Dangerous Crossroads.* Boston: South End Press, 1995:217–230.

————. L'anthropologue face à la pauvreté et au sida dans un contexte rural. In Benoist, J., Desclaux, A. (eds.). *Anthropologie et sida: Bilan et perspectives.* Paris: Editions Karthala, 1996:89–106.

————. Quelles possibilités de réponses locales face au nouvel ordre mondial? In Hurbon, L. (ed.). *Les Transitions démocratiques.* Paris: Syros, 1996:257–264.

————. Women, poverty, and AIDS. In Farmer, P. E., Connors, M., Simmons, J. (eds.). *Women, Poverty, and AIDS: Sex, Drugs, and Structural Violence.* Monroe, Maine: Common Courage Press, 1996:3–38.

————. Ethnography, social analysis, and the prevention of sexually transmitted HIV infection. In Inhorn, M., Brown, P. (eds.). *The Anthropology of Infectious Disease.* Amsterdam: Gordon and Breach, 1997:413–438.

————. AIDS and social scientists—Critical reflections. In Becker, C., Dozon, J. P., Obbo, C., Touré, M. (eds.). *Vivre et penser le sida en Afrique.* Paris: Editions Karthala, 1999:33–39.

————. Cruel and unusual: Drug-resistant tuberculosis as punishment. In Stern, V. (ed.). *Sentenced to Die? The Problem of TB in Prisons in East and Central Europe and Central Asia.* London: Prison Reform International, 1999:70–88.

————. Brujería, política, y concepciones sobre el sida en el Haití rural. In Armus, D. (ed.). *Entre Curanderos y Médicos: Historia, Cultura, y Enfermedad en América Latina.* Buenos Aires: Grupo Editorial Norma, 2002: 419–455.

————. AIDS e mazzismo: Medicina, stereotipi ed epidemiologia tra gli immigrati haitiani negli USA, 1981–1994. In *Spettri di Haiti: Dal colonialismo francese all'imperialismo americano.* Verona: OmbreCorte, 2002.

————. The house of the dead: Tuberculosis and incarceration. In Mauer, M., Chesney-Lind, M. (eds.). *Invisible Punishment: The Collateral Consequences of Mass Imprisonment.* New York: The New Press, 2002: 239–257.

Farmer, P. E., Bertrand, D. Hypocrisies of development: Health and health care among the Haitian rural poor. In Kim, J. Y., Millen, J. V., Gershman, J., Irwin, A. (eds.). *Dying for Growth: Global Inequalities and the Health of the Poor.* Monroe, Maine: Common Courage Press, 2000:65–90.

Farmer, P. E., Castro, A. Salud y derechos humanos: una vía para la medicina y la salud pública. In *Derechos humanos y salud: Encontrando los lazos.* Lima, Peru: Edhuca Salud, 2002:88–90.

Farmer, P. E., Connors, M., Fox, K., Furin, J. J. Rereading social science. In Farmer, P. E., Connors, M., Simmons, J. (eds.). *Women, Poverty, and AIDS: Sex, Drugs, and Structural Violence.* Monroe, Maine: Common Courage Press, 1996:147–205.

Farmer, P. E., Daily, J. Tuberculosis: Essentials of diagnosis, treatment, and prophylaxis. In Thaler, S. J., Maguire, J. H., Sax, P. E. (eds.). *Primary Care Handbook of Infectious Diseases.* Totowa, N.J.: Humana Press, in press.

Farmer, P. E., Good, B. Illness representations in medical anthropology: A critical review and a case study of the representation of AIDS in Haiti. In Skelton, J., Coryle, R. C. (eds.). *The Mental Representation of Health and Illness.* New York: Springer-Verlag, 1991:131–167.

Farmer, P. E., Kim, J. Y., Mitnick, C., Timperi, R. Responding to outbreaks of multidrug-resistant tuberculosis: Introducing "DOTS-Plus." In Reichman, L. B., Hershfield, E. S. (eds.). *Tuberculosis: A Comprehensive International Approach.* Second ed. New York: Marcel Dekker, 1999: 447–469.

Farmer, P. E., Shin, S. S., Bayona, J., Kim, J. Y., Furin, J. J., Brenner, J. G. Making DOTS-Plus work. In Bastian, I., Portaels, F. (eds.). *Tuberculosis.* Dordrecht, Netherlands: Kluwer Academic Publishers, 2000: 285–306.

Farmer, P. E., Walton, D. Condoms, coups, and the ideology of prevention: Facing failure in rural Haiti. In Keenan, J., Fuller, J., Cahill, L. S. (eds.). *Catholic Ethicists on HIV/AIDS Prevention.* New York and London: Continuum, 2000:108–119.

Farmer, P. E., Walton, D., Becerra, M. C. International tuberculosis control in the twenty-first century. In Friedman, L. N. (ed.). *Tuberculosis: Current Concepts and Treatment.* Boca Raton, Fla.: CRC Press, 2000:475–495.

Farmer, P. E., Walton, D. A., Furin, J. J. The changing face of AIDS: Implications for policy and practice. In Mayer, K. D., Pizer, H. F. (eds.). *The Emergence of AIDS: The Impact on Immunology, Microbiology, and Public Health.* Washington, D.C.: APHA, 2000:139–247.

Kim, J. Y., Shakow, A. Castro, A., Vanderwarker, C., Farmer, P. E. Specificity and collectivity of global public goods: The case of tuberculosis control. *In Global Public Goods for Health: Promoting Global Collective Action for Health.* Oxford: Oxford University Press, for the World Health Organization, in press.

Shin, S. S., Bayona, J., Farmer, P. E. DOTS and DOTS-Plus: Not the only answer. In Davies, P.D.O. (ed.) *Clinical Tuberculosis.* Third ed. London: Arnold Publishers, in press.

Simmons, J., Farmer, P. E., Schoepf, B. G. A global perspective. In Farmer, P. E., Connors, M., Simmons, J. (eds.). *Women, Poverty, and AIDS: Sex, Drugs, and Structural Violence.* Monroe, Maine: Common Courage Press, 1996:39–90.

Viaud, G., Farmer, P. E., Nicoleau, G. Haitian teens confront AIDS: A Partners In Health program on social justice and AIDS prevention. In Goldstein, N., Manlowe, J. (eds.). *The Gender Politics of HIV/AIDS in Women: Perspectives on the Pandemic in the U.S.* New York: New York University Press, 1997:302–322.

JOURNAL ARTICLES

Banatvala, N., Matic, S., Kimerling, M., Farmer, P. E., Goldfarb, A. Tuberculosis in Russia. *Lancet* 1999; 354:1036.

Becerra, M. C., Freeman, J., Bayona, J., Shin, S. S., Furin, J. J., Kim, J. Y., Werner, B., Timperi, R., Sloutsky, A., Wilson, M. E., Pagano, M., Farmer, P. E. Using treatment failure under effective directly observed short-course chemotherapy programs to identify patients with multidrug-resistant tuberculosis. *International Journal of Tuberculosis and Lung Disease* 2000; 4(2):108–114.

Castro, A., Farmer, P. E. Anthropologie de la violence: La culpabilisation des victimes. *Notre librairie: Revue des littératures du sud* 2002; 148:102–108.

Cohen, A., Farmer, P. E., Kleinman, A. Health-behaviour interventions: With whom? *Health Transition Review* 1997; 7:84–89.

Farmer, P. E., Haitians without a home. *Aeolus* (Duke University) Feb. 24, 1982.

―――. The anthropologist within. *Harvard Medical Alumni Bulletin* 1985; 59(1):23–28.

―――. Bad blood, spoiled milk: Body fluids as moral barometers in rural Haiti. *American Ethnologist* 1988; 15(1):62–83.

―――. Blood, sweat, and baseballs: Haiti in the West Atlantic system. *Dialectical Anthropology* 1988; 13(1):83–99.

―――. The exotic and the mundane: Human immunodeficiency virus in Haiti. *Human Nature* 1990; 1(4):415–446.

―――. Sending sickness: Sorcery, politics, and changing concepts of AIDS in rural Haiti. *Medical Anthropology Quarterly* 1990; 4(1):6–27.

―――. Pauvreté à risque. *Sidalerte* 1992; 18:24–25.

―――. The power of the poor in Haiti. *America* 1992; 164(9):260–267.

―――. Graham Greene: An appreciation from Haiti. *America* 1993; 168(4):17–20.

―――. AIDS-talk and the constitution of cultural models. *Social Science and Medicine* 1994; 38(6):801–809.

―――. What's at stake in Haiti? *Z Magazine* 1994; 7(2):21–25.

―――. Medicine and social justice. *America* 1995; 173(2):13–17.

―――. On suffering and structural violence: A view from below. *Daedalus* 1995; 125(1):261–283.

―――. Haiti's lost years: Lessons for the Americas. *Current Issues in Public Health* 1996; 2(3):143–151.

―――. Social inequalities and emerging infectious diseases. *Emerging Infectious Diseases* 1996; 2(4):259–269.

―――. AIDS and anthropologists: Ten years later. *Medical Anthropology Quarterly* 1997; 11(4):516–525.

―――. Letter from Haiti. *AIDS Clinical Care* 1997; 9(11):83–85.

―――. Listening for prophetic voices in medicine. *America* 1997; 177 (1):8–13.

―――. Social scientists and the new tuberculosis. *Social Science and Medicine* 1997; 44(3):347–358.

―――. Inequalities and antivirals. *Pharos* 1998; 61(2):34–38.

―――. A visit to Chiapas. *America* 1998; 178(10):14–18.

―――. Case 8, Clinicopathological Conferences: Gram-negative sepsis of uncertain etiology. *New England Journal of Medicine* 1999; 340(10):869–876.

―――. Desigualdades sociales y enfermedades infecciosas emergentes. *Tareas* 1999; (102):77–97.

―――. Hidden epidemics of tuberculosis. *Infectious Disease and Social Inequalities: From Hemispheric Insecurity to Global Cooperation.* A Working

Paper of the Latin American Program at the Woodrow Wilson International Center for Scholars. Washington, D.C.: Wilson Center, 1999; 31–55.

———. Managerial successes, clinical failures. *International Journal of Tuberculosis and Lung Disease* 1999; 3(5):365–367.

———. Pathologies of power: Rethinking health and human rights. *American Journal of Public Health* 1999; 89(10):1486–96.

———. TB superbugs: The coming plague on all our houses. *Natural History* 1999; 108(3):46–53.

———. The consumption of the poor: Tuberculosis in the twenty-first century. *Ethnography* 2000; 1(2):211–244.

———. The major infectious diseases in the world—to treat or not to treat? *New England Journal of Medicine* 2001; 345(3):208–210.

———. Can transnational research be ethical in the developing world? *Lancet* 2002; 360:1266.

Farmer, P. E., Bayona, J., Becerra, M. Multidrug-resistant tuberculosis and the need for biosocial perspectives. *International Journal of Tuberculosis and Lung Disease* 2001; 5(10):885–886.

Farmer, P. E., Bayona, J., Becerra, M., Furin, J. J., Henry, C., Hiatt, H., Kim, J. Y., Mitnick, C. D., Nardell, E., Shin, S. S. The dilemma of MDRTB in the global era. *International Journal of Tuberculosis and Lung Disease* 1998; 2(11):869–876.

Farmer, P. E., Bayona, J., Becerra, M., Kim, J. Y., Shin, S. S. Reducing transmission through community-based treatment of multidrug-resistant tuberculosis. *International Journal of Tuberculosis and Lung Disease* 1998; 2(11 supp. 2):S190.

Farmer, P. E., Bayona, J., Shin, S. S., Alvarez, L., Becerra, M., Nardell, E., Nuñez, C., Sanchez, E., Timperi, R., Kim, J. Y. Preliminary results of community-based MDRTB treatment in Lima, Peru. *International Journal of Tuberculosis and Lung Disease* 1998; 2(11 supp. 2):S371.

Farmer, P. E., Furin, J. J. Sexe, drogue, et violences structurelles: Les femmes et le V.I.H. *Journal des Anthropologues* 1997; 68–69:35–46.

Farmer, P. E., Furin, J. J., Bayona, J., Becerra, M., Henry, C., Hiatt, H., Kim, J. Y., Mitnick, C. D., Nardell, E., Shin, S. S. Management of MDR-TB in resource-poor countries. *International Journal of Tuberculosis and Lung Disease* 1999; 3(8):643–645.

Farmer, P. E., Furin, J. J., Shin, S. S. Managing multidrug-resistant tuberculosis. *Journal of Respiratory Diseases* 2000; 21(1):53–56.

Farmer, P. E., Gastineau, N. Rethinking health and human rights: Time for a paradigm shift. *The Journal of Law, Medicine & Ethics* 2002; 30(4):655–666.

Farmer, P. E., Kim, J. Y. Anthropology, accountability, and the prevention of AIDS. *Journal of Sex Research* 1991; 25(2):203–221.

———. Community-based approaches to the control of multidrug-resistant tuberculosis: Introducing "DOTS-plus." *British Medical Journal* 1998; 317:671–674.

———. Resurgent TB in Russia: Do we know enough to act? *European Journal of Public Health* 2000; 10(2):150–152.

Farmer, P. E., Kleinman, A. AIDS as human suffering. *Daedalus* 1989; 118(2):135–160.

Farmer, P. E., Léandre, F., Mukherjee, J. S., Claude, M. S., Nevil, P., Smith-Fawzi, M. C., Koenig, S. P., Castro, A., Becerra, M. C., Sachs, J., Attaran, A., Kim, J. Y. Community-based approaches to HIV treatment in resource-poor settings. *Lancet* 2001; 358:404–409.

Farmer, P. E., Léandre, F., Mukherjee, J., Gupta, R., Tarter, L., Kim, J. Y. Community-based treatment of advanced HIV disease: Introducing DOT-HAART (directly observed therapy with highly active antiretroviral therapy). *WHO Bulletin* 2001; 79(12):1145–51.

Farmer, P. E., Lindenbaum, S., Good, M. J. Women, poverty, and AIDS: An introduction. *Culture, Medicine, and Psychiatry* 1993; 17(4):387–398.

Farmer, P. E., Nardell, E. Nihilism and pragmatism in tuberculosis control. *American Journal of Public Health* 1998; 88(7):4–5.

Farmer, P. E., Robin, S., Ramilus, S. L., Kim, J. Y. Tuberculosis, poverty, and "compliance": Lessons from rural Haiti. *Seminars in Respiratory Infections* 1991; 6(4):254–260.

Farmer, P. E., Rylko-Bauer, B. L. L'exceptionnel système de santé américain: Critique d'une médecine à vocation commerciale. *Actes de la recherche en Sciences sociales* 2001; 139:13–30.

Farmer, P. E., Smith-Fawzi, M. C., Nevil, P. Unjust embargo of aid for Haiti. *Lancet* 2003; 361:420–423.

Farmer, P. E., Walton, D., Tarter, L. Infections and inequalities. *Global Change and Human Health* 2000; 1(2):94–109.

Furin, J. J., Mitnick, C., Shin, S. S., Bayona, J., Becerra, M., Singler, J., Alcántara, F., Castaneda, C., Sánchez, E., Acha, J., Farmer, P. E., Kim, J. Y. Occurrence of serious adverse effects in patients receiving community-based therapy for multidrug-resistant tuberculosis. *International Journal for Tuberculosis and Lung Disease* 2001; 5(7):648–654.

Furin, J. J., Becerra, M. C., Shin, S. S., Kim, J. Y., Bayona, J., Farmer, P. E. Effect of administering short-course, standard regimens in individuals infected with drug-resistant *Mycobacterium tuberculosis* strains. *European Journal of Clinical Microbiology and Infectious Diseases* 2000; 19(1):132–136.

Furin, J. J., Mitnick, C. D., Becerra, M., Shin, S. S., Singler, J. M., Bayona, J., Alcántara, F., Sánchez, E., Bomann, M., Kim, J. Y., Farmer, P. E. Absence of serious adverse effects in a cohort of Peruvian patients receiving community-based treatment for multidrug-resistant tuberculosis (MDR-TB). *International Journal of Tuberculosis and Lung Disease* 1999; 3(9 supp. 1):S81.

Gaines, A., Farmer, P. E. Visible saints: Social cynosures and dysphoria in the Mediterranean tradition. *Culture, Medicine, and Psychiatry* 1986; 10(4):295–330.

Gupta, R., Kim, J. Y., Espinal, M. A., Caudron, J.-M., Pecoul, B., Farmer, P. E., Raviglione, M. C. Responding to market failures in tuberculosis control. *Science* 2001; 293:1049–51.

Kim, J. Y., Furin, J. J., Shakow, A. D., Millen, J. V., Brenner, J. G., Fordyce, M. W., Lyon, E., Bayona, J., Farmer, P. E. Treatment of multidrug-resistant tuberculosis (MDR-TB): New strategies for procuring second-and third-line drugs. *International Journal of Tuberculosis and Lung Disease* 1999; 3(9 supp. 1):S81.

Miranda, J., Farmer, P. E. Social exclusion must be considered in global terms. *British Medical Journal* 2001; 323:1370.

Mitnick, C., Bayona, J., Palacios, E., Shin, S. S., Furin, J. J., Alcántara, F., Sánchez, E., Sarria, M., Becerra, M., Smith-Fawzi, M. C., Kapiga, S., Neuberg, D., Maguire, J. H., Kim, J. Y., Farmer, P. E. Community-based therapy for multidrug-resistant tuberculosis in Lima, Peru. *New England Journal of Medicine* 2003; 348(2):119–128.

Mukherjee, J. S., Shin, S. S., Furin, J. J., Rich, M. L., Léandre, F., Joseph, K. J., Seung, K., Acha, J., Gelmanova, I., Goncharova, E., Pasechnikov, A., Virú, F. A., Farmer, P. E. New challenges in the clinical management of drug-resistant tuberculosis. *Infectious Diseases in Clinical Practice,* in press.

Rylko-Bauer, B., Farmer, P. E. Managed care or managed inequality? A call for critiques of market-based medicine. *Medical Anthropology Quarterly* 2002; 16(4):476–502.

Singler, J., Farmer, P. E. Treating HIV in resource-poor settings. *MSJAMA* 2002; 288:1652–1653.

Timperi, R., Sloutsky, A., Farmer, P. E. Global laboratory testing capacity for tuberculosis. *International Journal of Tuberculosis and Lung Disease* 1998; 2(11 supp. 2):S290–291.

OTHER

Farmer, P. E. Social medicine and the challenge of bio-social research. In Innovative Structures in Basic Research: Ringberg-Symposium 4–7 October 2000. Plehn, G. (ed.). Munich: Generalverwaltung der Max-Planck-Gesellschaft, Referat für Presse- und Öffentlichkeitsarbeit, pp. 55–73. Available at http://www.mpiwg-berlin.mpg.de/ringberg/main.html.

———. Prevention without treatment is not sustainable. *National AIDS Bulletin* (Australia) 2000; 13(6):6–9, 40.

———. What is appropriate empiric therapy for active tuberculosis? Ask the Expert. *APUA Newsletter* 2000; 18(3):6.

———. AIDS heretic. *New Internationalist* Jan.–Feb. 2001; 331:14–16.

———. Arresting global epidemics: Are some people too poor to treat? *GSAS Newsletter* (Harvard University) 2001: 4–5, 12–13.

———. Use of antiretroviral therapy in developing countries: A biosocial analysis. Abstracts of the 10th Conference on Retroviruses and Opportunistic Infections, Boston, 2003, session 92, abstract 48, p. 4.

Farmer, P. E., Castro, A. Un pilote en Haïti: De l'efficacité de la distribution d'antiviraux dans des pays pauvres, et des objections qui lui sont faites. *Vacarme* Apr. 2002; 19:17–22.

———. Castigo a los más pobres de América. *El País,* Jan. 12, 2003, p. 8–9.

———. Urgence humanitaire en Haiti. *Courrier International* 2003; 640:20–21.

Farmer, P. E., Léandre, F., Bayona, J., Louissaint, M. DOTS-Plus for the poorest of the poor: The Partners In Health experience in Haiti. *International Journal of Tuberculosis and Lung Disease* 2001; 5(11):S257.

Farmer, P. E., Léandre, F., Koenig, S. P., Nevil, P. Mukherjee, J., Ferrer, J., Walker, B., Orélus, C., Smith-Fawzi, M. C. Preliminary outcomes of directly observed treatment of advanced HIV disease with ARVs (DOT-HAART) in rural Haiti. Abstracts of the 10th Conference on Retroviruses and Opportunistic Infections, Boston, 2003, session 33, abstract 171, p. 120.

Naroditskaya, V., Werner, B. G., Farmer, P. E., Becerra, M., Sloutsky, A. Limited mutation pattern found by DNA sequence analysis of rifampin-resistant (rif-R) clinical Mycobacterium tuberculosis isolates from Peru. Abstracts of the Annual Meeting of the American Society of Microbiology, Chicago, Ill., 1999, session 27U, abstract U-11, p. 635.

Walton, D., Farmer, P. E. The new white plague. *MSJAMA* (online), 2000, 284(21):2789.

I found the following materials on Haiti especially useful:
Aristide, J.-B. *In the Parish of the Poor.* Maryknoll, N.Y.: Orbis Books, 1990.

Bell, M. S. *All Souls Rising*. New York: Pantheon, 1995.

―――. *Master of the Crossroads*. New York: Pantheon, 2005.

Danner, M. Beyond the mountains I. *New Yorker,* Nov. 27, 1989, pp. 55–100.

Gaillard, R. *Hinche Mise en Croix*. Port-au-Prince, Haiti: Imprimerie Le Natal, 1982.

Greene, G. *The Comedians*. London: Bodley Head, 1966.

Hall, R. A., Jr. *Haitian Creole: Grammar, Texts, Vocabulary*. Philadelphia: American Folklore Society, 1953.

Heinl, R. B., Jr., and Heinl, N. G., rev. by Heinl, M. *Written in Blood: The Story of the Haitian People, 1492–1995*. Lanham, Md.: University Press of America, 1996.

James, C.L.R. *The Black Jacobins: Touissant Louverture and the San Domingo Revolution*. Second ed. New York: Vintage Books, 1989.

Métraux, A., trans. by Hugo Charteris. *Voodoo in Haiti*. New York: Schocken Books, 1972.

Shacochis, B. *The Immaculate Invasion*. New York: Viking Press, 1999.

Wilentz, A. *The Rainy Season: Haiti After Duvalier*. New York: Simon and Schuster, 1989.

Books and journal articles about tuberculosis and AIDS could fill an entire library. For the reader interested in the clinical and sociological literature on those diseases, I recommend Farmer's works and the material cited in his footnotes and bibliographies. I also recommend the following books and their cited references:

Bukhman, G. *Reform and Resistance in Post-Soviet Tuberculosis Control*. Doctoral diss., University of Arizona, Tucson. Ann Arbor: University Microfilms, 2001.

Garrett, L. *The Coming Plague: Newly Emerging Diseases in a World out of Balance*. New York: Farrar, Straus and Giroux, 1994.

―――. *Betrayal of Trust: The Collapse of Global Public Health*. New York: Hyperion, 2000.

I used the following as an introduction to the history of cost-effectiveness analysis:

Shakow, A. *A Brief History of Cost Efficacy*. Working paper, Partners In Health, Boston, 2000.

An influential example of cost-effectiveness analysis applied to tuberculosis control can be found in the following:

Murray, C.J.L., DeJonghe, E., Chum, H. J., Nyangulu, D. S., Salomao, A., Styblo, K. Cost effectiveness of chemotherapy for pulmonary tuberculosis in three sub-Saharan African countries. *Lancet* 1991; 338: 1305–1308.

The first quotation from WHO, in Chapter 15 of this book, comes from:
World Health Organization, *Treatment of Tuberculosis: Guidelines for National Programmes.* Second edition. Geneva, 1997.

The second quotation comes from:
World Health Organization, *Groups at Risk: WHO Report on the Tuberculosis Epidemic.* Geneva, 1998.

Note also this quotation: "The WHO Tuberculosis Programme has recommended that treatment of chronic cases with [second-line] drugs remain a low priority for national tuberculosis programmes in developing countries due to their high costs and the limited prospects for cure of those cases."
Weil, D. Drug supply—Meeting a global need. In *Tuberculosis: Back to the Future.* Porter, J., McAdam, K. (eds.). Chichester: John Wiley, 1994, 124–129; quoted in Farmer, *Infections and Inequalities.*

For information on New York City's epidemic, the following journal articles provide a good beginning:
Brudney, K., Dobkin, J. Resurgent tuberculosis in New York City: Human immunodeficiency virus, homelessness, and the decline of tuberculosis control programs. *American Review of Respiratory Disease* 1991; 144:745–749.
Frieden, T. R., Fujiwara, E., Washko, R., Hamburg, M. Tuberculosis in New York City: Turning the tide. *New England Journal of Medicine* 1995; 333(4):229–233.

A fine overview of the TB epidemic in Russia can be found in the report assembled by Partners In Health:
The Global Impact of Drug-Resistant Tuberculosis. Boston: Program in Infectious Disease and Social Change, Department of Social Medicine, Harvard Medical School, 1999.

I also made use of this book on MDR-TB:
Reichman, L. B., with Tanne, J. H. *Timebomb: The Global Epidemic of Multi-Drug-Resistant Tuberculosis.* New York: McGraw-Hill, 2002.

Farmer's works and the books by Bukhman, Garrett, and Reichman offer useful views of international health. I also relied on the following:

Kim, J. Y., Millen, J. V., Irwin, A., Gershman, J. (eds.). *Dying for Growth: Global Inequality and the Health of the Poor.* Monroe, Maine: Common Courage Press, 2000.

Muraskin, W. *The Politics of International Health: The Children's Vaccine Initiative and the Struggle to Develop Vaccines for the Third World.* Albany: State University of New York Press, 1998.

For my description of Rudolf Virchow's work, I used the following:

Ackerknecht, E. H. *Rudolph Virchow: Doctor, Statesman, Anthropologist.* Madison: University of Wisconsin, 1953.

Boyd, B. A. *Rudolph Virchow: The Scientist as Citizen.* New York and London: Garland, 1991.

Eisenberg, L. Rudolf Ludwig Karl Virchow, where are you now that we need you? *American Journal of Medicine* 1984; 77(3):524–532.

Also this odd but rather wonderful source:

Rudolph Virchow on Pathology Education. Lecture by "Ed" at a meeting of the Group for Research in Pathology Education, Hershey, Pa. (To be found on the website www.pathguy.com/lectures/virchow.htm.)

The material on Mother Teresa comes from

Hitchens, C. *The Missionary Position.* London and New York: Verso, 1995.

Cuba's AIDS sanitorium was called a concentration camp in the following op-ed article:

Rosenthal, A. M. Individual ethics and the plague. *New York Times,* May 26, 1987, sec. A, p. 23.

For a temperate account of Cuba's AIDS policy, and an accurate description of Santiago de las Vegas, I recommend the following article:

Scheper-Hughes, N. AIDS, public health, and human rights in Cuba. *Lancet* 1993; 342:965–967

For Farmer's full comparison of the two AIDS quarantines in Cuba, see his Pathologies of Power.

For a fascinating article on Peru and its civil war, I recommend:

Starn, O. Missing the revolution: Anthropologists and the war in Peru. In

Rereading Cultural Anthropology. Marcus, G. (ed.). Durham, N.C.: Duke University Press, 1992.

The newspaper article cited in regard to Alex Goldfarb is:
Gill, P. Russian defector fears for life. *Russia Journal Weekly,* Nov. 11, 2000.

See also:
Reichman, *Timebomb,* and Gessen, M. From Russia with secrets: What will he expose? *U.S. News and World Report,* Nov. 13, 2000.

For more information about Partners in Health, go to www.pih.org.

Mountains Beyond Mountains

_____

Tracy Kidder

A Reader's Guide

To print out copies of this or other
Random House Reader's Guides,
visit us at www.atrandom.com/rgg

Questions for Discussion

1. Paul Farmer finds ways of connecting with people whose backgrounds are vastly different from his own. How does he do this? Are his methods something to which we can all aspire?

2. Paul Farmer believes that "if you're making sacrifices . . . you're trying to lessen some psychic discomfort" (p. 24). Do you agree with the way that Farmer makes personal sacrifices? For what kinds of things do you make sacrifices, and when do you expect others to make them?

3. Kidder points out that Farmer is dissatisfied with the current distribution of money and medicine in the world. What is your opinion of the distribution of these forms of wealth? What would you change, if you could?

4. Farmer designed a study to find out whether there was a correlation between his Haitian patients' belief in sorcery as the cause of TB and their recovery from that disease through medical treatment. What did he discover about the relative importance of cultural beliefs among his impoverished patients and their material circumstances? Do you think that this discovery might have broad application—for instance, to situations in the United States?

5. The title of the book comes from the Haitian proverb, "Beyond mountains there are mountains." What does the saying mean in the context of the culture it comes from, and what does it mean in relation to Farmer's work? Can you think of other situations—personal or societal—for which this proverb might be apt?

6. Paul Farmer had an eccentric childhood, and his accomplishments have been unique. Do you see a correlation between the way Farmer was raised and how he has chosen to live his life? How has your own background influenced your life and your decisions?

7. Compare Zanmi Lasante to the Socios en Salud project in Carabayllo. Consider how the projects got started, the relationships between doctors and patients, and the involvement of the international community.

8. Kidder explains that Farmer and his colleagues at PIH were asked by some academics, "Why do you call your patients poor people? They don't call themselves poor people" (p. 100). How do Farmer and Jim Kim confront the issue of how to speak honestly about the people they work to help? How do they learn to speak honestly with each other, and what is the importance of the code words and acronyms that they share (for example, AMC's, or Areas of Moral Clarity)?

9. Ophelia Dahl and Tom White both play critical roles in this book and in the story of Partners In Health. How are their acts of compassion different from Farmer's?

10. Tracy Kidder has written elsewhere that the choice of point of view is the most important an author makes in constructing a work of narrative nonfiction. He has also written that finding a point of view that works is a matter of making a choice among tools, and that the choice should be determined not by theory, but by an author's immersion in the materials of the story itself. Kidder has never before written a book in which he made himself a character. Can you think of some of the reasons he might have had for doing this in *Mountains Beyond Mountains*?